walking**FIT**

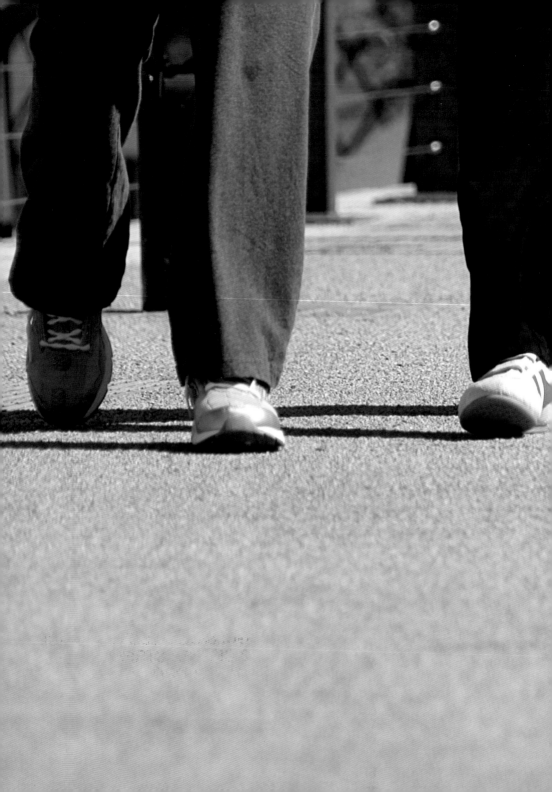

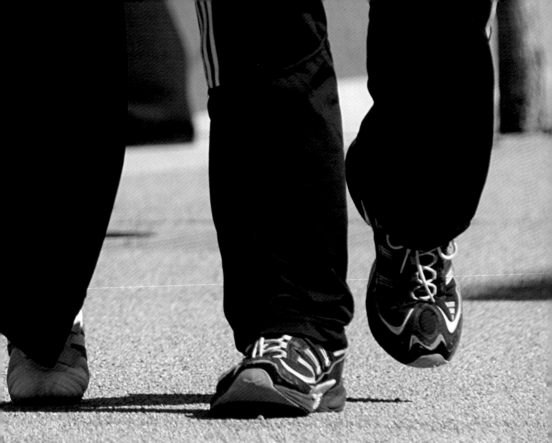

walking**FIT**

Rose Leach

COLLINS & BROWN

For my father, David, for being a genius.
For my mother, Patricia, and sister, Fleur, for being the greatest.

First published in Great Britain in 2005 by
Collins & Brown
The Chrysalis Building
Bramley Road
London W10 6SP

An imprint of **Chrysalis** Books Group plc

10 9 8 7 6 5 4 3 2 1

British Library Cataloguing-in-Publication Data:
A catalogue record for this book is available from the British Library.

ISBN 1 84340 312 9

Commissioning Editor: Victoria Alers-Hankey
Editor: Fiona Screen
Photographs: Guy Hearn
Design: Simon Daley
Models: Rose Leach, Carly Madden, Rupert Barclay, Simon Briggs, Trudy Thomson,
Caroline de Albuquerque and Andrew Alers-Hankey

Reproduction by Classicscan PTE Ltd, Singapore
Printed and bound by CT Printing Ltd

The information, advice and exercises set out in this book are only a guide and not intended to cause injury if followed correctly. You should consult your doctor before beginning any fitness regime. The author and publisher disclaim any liability from and in connection with use of the information contained within this book.

Acknowledgements
Thanks to all the WOW! pioneers who believed in what we were doing and for inspiring us with their encouragement and enthusiasm. Thanks especially to Marc, Tina, Nikki, Anne-Mette, Trudy, Jill, Joanne, Margaret, Sally, Bina, Kim, Di, Bernadette and everyone at Healthy Lansbury.

Thanks to Victoria for all your support in writing this book, and to my mother and father, Tina, Tim F, Tim B, Trudy and Simon for your invaluable and varied input. Fleur, as always, you've been amazing. And thanks to Ben, Roly and Harry for keeping us walking whatever the weather!

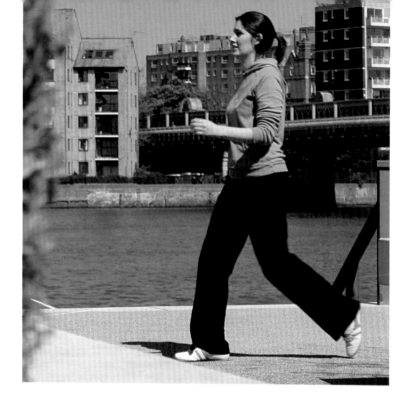

Contents

Introduction

According to the World Health Organisation, a low level of physical activity is now one of the ten leading global causes of serious illness, and is responsible for two million deaths worldwide each year. If you don't want to become one of these statistics, get active with us today.

What are your reasons for opening this book? Perhaps you would like to get fit, lose weight, have more energy or maybe you're just curious about the next health/fitness/diet approach? Whatever your reasons, you are about to discover a tried and tested formula that will open the door to a new, positive, turbo-charged phase of your life. It is called The Workout Walking (WOW!) Plan and you will be amazed by the results.

Start by reading the innovative yet straightforward ideas in Chapters 1–3 of this book and then follow the simple steps in The Workout Walking (WOW!) Plan (Chapter 4). In six weeks you will be well on your way to fulfilling your potential and striding towards the life you have always dreamed of. This is not an empty promise – throughout *Walking Fit* you will read about people whose lives have changed for the better thanks to The WOW! Plan. The plan has succeeded time and again, helping people to:

- ▶ Get fit.
- ▶ Lose weight (and, more importantly, lose inches).
- ▶ Tone up and improve muscle tone.
- ▶ Improve existing medical conditions and increase resistance to disease.
- ▶ Boost energy levels.
- ▶ Heighten spirits and reduce depression.
- ▶ Raise self-esteem and confidence.
- ▶ Sleep better.
- ▶ Get outside in the fresh air, see the sights and make friends!

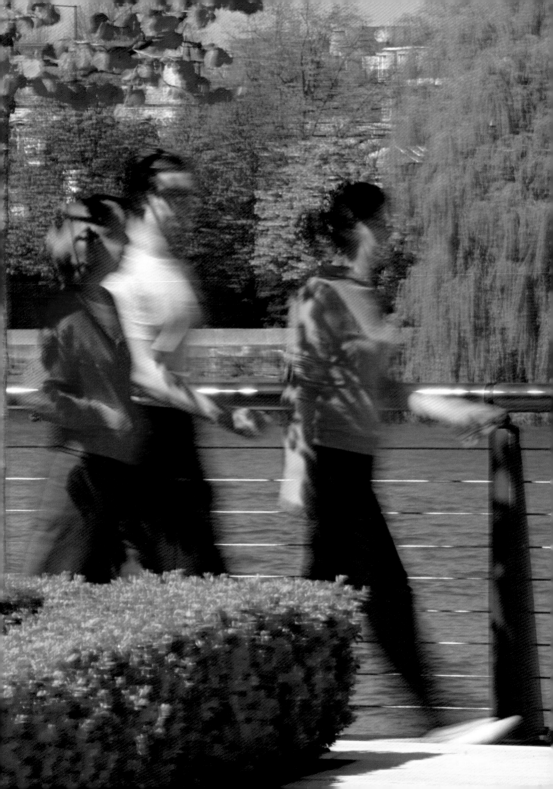

The WOW! Plan provides a positive, enjoyable antidote to the doom and gloom we are confronted with on a daily basis about the poor state of our collective health. The number of people in the Western world suffering from obesity and diseases such as diabetes, heart disease and cancer has rocketed in recent years. This is primarily down to three factors: physical inactivity, poor eating habits and stress. But you can help to turn this situation around.

Living a happy and healthy life is not easy. Our lives have become overly complicated and stressful with an abundance of choices and general information overload. We are inundated with both time- and labour-saving 'solutions' designed to make our lives more comfortable and instantly gratifying. In the process, our bodies and minds are suffering from lack of use, overuse or misuse.

In *Walking Fit* you will be shown how to get more from walking, by using your body in different ways and so maximising the impact on your heart, lungs and muscles. And you'll begin to understand how eating the right foods will give you the energy and drive to get the most out of your exercise and daily life.

CASE STUDY **Trudy (38)**

Joining Workout Walking (WOW!) was an incredible insight into my own health and fitness levels and a solution to help me improve. Since joining Rose and Marc in January 2004, my lifestyle has completely changed. My car is no longer used on a daily basis as I walk just about everywhere. I save money by hardly needing to use public transport as I now tend to walk to reach my destinations. I have enjoyed walking around my city and discovering places and streets I never knew existed. I have lost 27kg (60lbs) since starting The WOW! Plan 12 months ago and my overall fitness levels have improved. It has made walking fun, sociable and an excellent way for me to keep positive and increase my self-esteem.

Many people have already benefited from the power of The WOW! Plan and the results have been staggering. By using some of their time each day to go walking, and by making simple changes to their diet, they have all experienced an improvement in their daily lives, including feeling calmer, younger, fitter and happier. Not only that, but they have been kept going by the fact that they have more energy, more confidence and a brighter outlook.

This is not a fad. The WOW! Plan has been shown to work time and again, and all it takes is the ability to walk and the desire to make positive changes in your life. This book will show you the rest. The WOW! Plan has been successful because:

- ▶ **It offers something entirely new, that WORKS.**
- ▶ **There are no hefty gym fees or fancy clothing or equipment, just yourself and a desire to become happier and healthier.**
- ▶ **It fits easily into any lifestyle, however busy.**
- ▶ **It can be done by almost anyone, anywhere.**
- ▶ **It provides PERMANENT results by helping you make simple yet highly effective long-term changes in your life.**

Read this book and set yourself free from ill health, tiredness, depression and the four walls surrounding you right now. You'll find that if you get the basics right you don't need complicated or expensive solutions.

How to use this book

Walking Fit has been made as easy as possible to read and use. The aim is to get you out there walking right away, so only essential, relevant information is included, with a healthy dose of motivation and inspiration!

Start right (Chapter 1) is designed to get you off on the right foot and ensure that everything you do makes a positive difference to your life, not just now, but permanently. Key to this is learning to behave like a successful person, from an athlete to a managing director, by setting

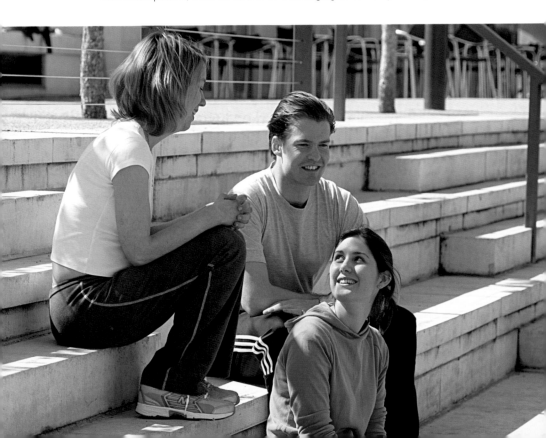

SMART goals (see page 25). These goals will keep you focused at all times on what you're doing and why. This simple exercise will make the difference between failure and success.

Clothing & equipment (Chapter 2) will give you some helpful hints on how to dress for both summer and winter walking, and introduce you to some gadgets that will help you measure your progress and keep you moving as fast as you would like.

Eating & exercise (Chapter 3) provides useful information on how best to maximise your energy both for walking and throughout the day, by fuelling your body with the right foods (and drinks).

The Workout Walking (WOW!) Plan (Chapter 4) gets down to business with your 6-week plan. Each week is broken into three areas: Daily targets, Walking Plan and Eating Plan. In each of the 6 weeks you'll be introduced to new physical activity targets.

This chapter introduces you to six highly successful Workout Walking (WOW!) techniques that will transform forever the way you view walking and its benefits, and includes advice on breathing and how to avoid bad posture when walking normally. The Eating Plan gives you three new nutritional tasks each week.

Finally, find out how you can test yourself and monitor how far and fast you're progressing in **Having fun** (Chapter 5). There are some great ideas here on how to maximise your enjoyment of walking.

Throughout, you will be reminded to focus on why you have chosen *Walking Fit*, and motivated with regular progress reports on how far you've walked and how many calories you've burned off. It's all right here – so enjoy!

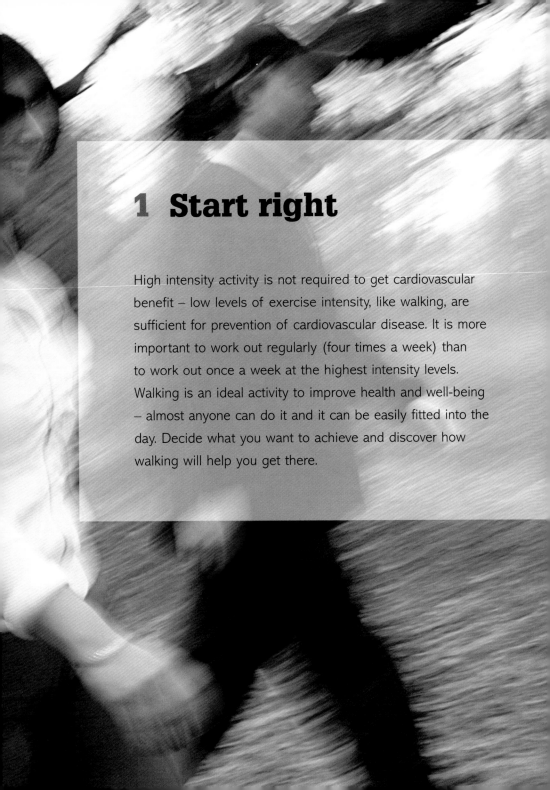

1 Start right

High intensity activity is not required to get cardiovascular benefit – low levels of exercise intensity, like walking, are sufficient for prevention of cardiovascular disease. It is more important to work out regularly (four times a week) than to work out once a week at the highest intensity levels. Walking is an ideal activity to improve health and well-being – almost anyone can do it and it can be easily fitted into the day. Decide what you want to achieve and discover how walking will help you get there.

Why walk?

Walking has often been described as the perfect exercise because it strengthens your heart, muscles and bones, keeps you flexible, and can stave off illness. Anyone who can walk can enjoy wide-ranging and very powerful benefits. It is simply not necessary to put your body under strain and risk injury in order to get fit, improve your health and raise your spirits – walking will do all this for you.

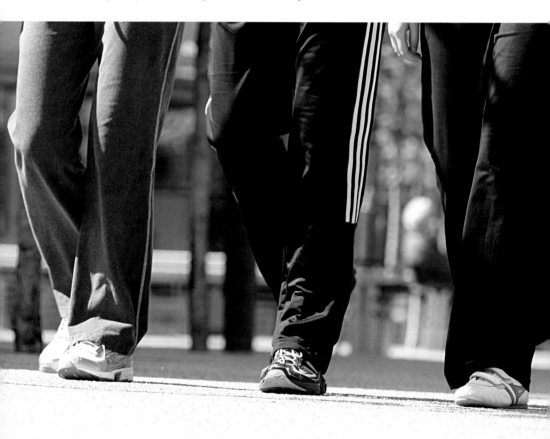

Physical and mental benefits aside, walking also offers the opportunity to get outside in the open air, meet new people, and discover new places only accessible on foot. You'd be amazed at some of the surprises right around the corner from where you live or work.

Decide today to make walking a part of your daily life and you will start reaping rewards right away.

Walking has recently enjoyed a great surge in popularity, with people realising how much fun it can be and what an ideal way it is of becoming fit and improving health. If you're still a sceptic, let us put to rest a few common misconceptions:

► Walking isn't enough to make you fit.
Wrong.
Walking makes you stronger, fitter and healthier by increasing your heart rate. It is also low impact, which means there is less risk of the injuries associated with other forms of exercise.

► Walking is only for older people who can't do other forms of exercise.
Wrong.
Anyone, regardless of gender, age or fitness level, can benefit from walking.

► Walking cannot help you lose weight.
Wrong again.
Walking is one of the best ways to lose weight, enabling you to shed the pounds from all over your body, including your upper body. Walking requires a greater range of movement than running.

'Moderate exercise – such as walking – is more likely to benefit people than short, high impact bursts in places such as gyms.'
NORWICH UNION HEALTHCARE'S ONLINE MAGAZINE NOV 2001

Who can benefit from walking?

Walking is a suitable and beneficial form of exercise for everyone, including people who, for health reasons are unable to practice other sports or rigorous forms of exercise. It provides the cardiovascular and other classic health benefits associated with more strenuous exercise such as running or cycling while being very low risk. Of course, as with any new exercise programme, you should talk to your doctor first, particularly if you are overweight, suffer chest pains when active, have an existing medical condition or have not exercised before.

Walking and the overweight or obese

'Studies have shown that walkers travelling at more than 5 miles an hour actually burn twice as many calories as runners going the same speed.'

JOURNAL OF SPORTS MEDICINE AND PHYSICAL FITNESS, DEC 2000

Obesity is linked to a variety of illnesses and diseases including heart disease, cancer and diabetes: if you are overweight or obese and would like to enjoy a longer, happier and healthier life, start walking today.

Walking is the perfect way to help you drop the excess pounds, allowing you to do it safely, without putting too much pressure on your heart, joints or muscles. You can dictate the pace. It is essential, though, that you take it gently when you start off. If you become out of breath or find it hard to carry on a conversation, that's a sign that you are pushing yourself too hard. Slow down or stop until you have recovered.

As your body works off excess weight and shrinks in size, increase the distance that you walk, then start to walk faster and eventually move on to walking up and down hills. Again, remember that if you become breathless or unable to talk comfortably you should slow down or return to level ground to prevent putting undue strain on your body. You will build up your fitness, stamina and heart health sooner than you think, becoming lighter and happier in the process.

Walking and heart disease

> '37% of Coronary Heart Disease (CHD) deaths are related to inactivity as compared to only 19% of CHD deaths being related to smoking.'
>
> WWW.BHFACTIVE.ORG.UK

Exercise, and in particular walking, can not only help people recover from heart disease, but also aid in its prevention. In the past, rest was prescribed for those recovering from serious heart problems.

Cholesterol – quick facts

High density lipoprotein (HDL) = 'good' cholesterol
Low density lipoprotein (LDL) = 'bad' cholesterol

▶ **Problem** Cholesterol becomes a problem when we have too much LDL that clogs our veins and arteries, increasing our risk of heart attacks and strokes.

▶ **Cause** Eating too much saturated fat, such as fatty meat, full-cream dairy products and certain vegetable oils, such as palm oil, coconut oil and hardened fats.

▶ **Solution** Plenty of exercise; including lots of fresh vegetables, fruit and cereals (which contain no cholesterol) in your diet; reducing your intake of foods that are high in cholesterol and saturated fats.

However, the most recent research now shows that exercise is good even for a heart that has already been damaged. Exercising increases blood flow to the heart, strengthening it in the process so that it pumps more blood with less effort. Exercising the heart can also help achieve and maintain a healthy weight and control diabetes, high blood pressure and high blood cholesterol, all of which are CHD risk factors. It also helps to reduce stress, increase energy levels and reduce pain.

Walking and pregnancy

It is important to exercise gently while pregnant, preferably for about 30 minutes at least 3–4 times a week. Do speak to your doctor before embarking on any exercise routine, but barring any unusual circumstances you will probably find that s/he recommends walking as an ideal form of aerobic exercise.

Walking before and after pregnancy can provide a wide range of benefits including:

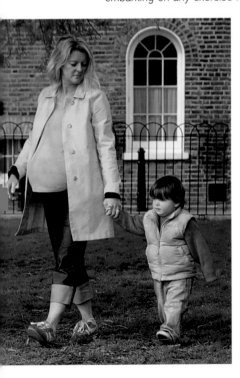

▶ Increased energy.
▶ Increased muscle tone, stamina and strength, making you better able to cope with the physical stress of labour and birth.
▶ Boosted circulation.
▶ Reduced stress.
▶ Reduced backache, constipation, tiredness and swelling.
▶ Better sleep.
▶ Ability to control your weight beforehand and aiding in weight loss after the birth.
▶ Keeping the 'baby blues' at bay following the birth by raising your spirits.

If you have not exercised before, start very slowly. If you are used to exercising, you may need to slow down during pregnancy. If you feel any pain, shortness of breath or excessive tiredness, slow down or stop. It is important that you don't overdo it and put your body and unborn baby under undue stress. Remember to keep hydrated at all times.

Walking and diabetes

Walking can be beneficial to diabetics by helping to regulate blood sugar levels and improve common symptoms such as excess body weight, high blood pressure and high cholesterol.

Diabetes occurs when the delicate balance of sugar (glucose) and insulin in the body is upset. Glucose, which we get from food, gives us energy and insulin is a substance secreted by the pancreas which removes any excess glucose from the bloodstream and stores it in the liver as glycogen. When glucose levels rise after eating or drinking, diabetes can occur if the pancreas is unable to produce enough extra insulin to maintain this balance.

If you suffer from diabetes, it is important that you prepare before starting an exercise programme. Your insulin requirements may change when you start exercising, so consult your doctor beforehand to discuss any required change in your medication. Ensure that you keep hydrated when you exercise: drink a large glass or water about 1 hour before you go for a walk and keep drinking small amounts at regular intervals during your session. Take a snack with you in case your blood sugar levels fall too low while you're out – symptoms of low blood sugar include a feeling of dizziness, nausea, lack of energy and blurred vision, and are often called a 'hypo'. The best time to exercise is about 2 hours after a meal, once your blood sugar levels have evened out after eating. When you return from your walk, you may need to eat a carbohydrate snack if your blood sugar levels have fallen too low.

Most importantly, monitor your body and how it's responding throughout your walk. With practise you will be able to fine-tune your preparations and concentrate on getting the most out of your workout.

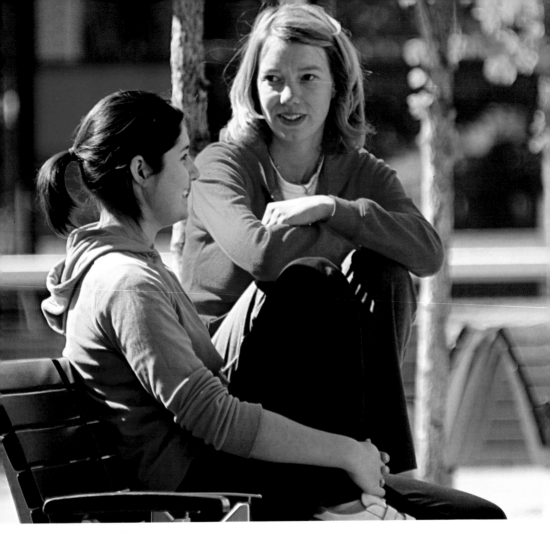

Walking and well-being

While most of us are keenly aware of the physical benefits of exercising, the powerful effects that exercise can have on our mental well-being are far less known. Mental health problems include anxiety, depression, post-natal depression, post-traumatic stress disorder and eating disorders. Ever-increasing numbers of people are being treated for these health problems. In fact, the state of our mental health is rapidly becoming one of the most serious global health issues: the World Health Organisation predicts that by 2020 depression will be second only to heart disease as an international health burden.

Recent studies have shown that exercise can play an important role in not only improving but also preventing mild to moderate depression – mounting evidence suggests that supervised, regular exercise such as walking can be as effective at alleviating common mental health problems as medication.

> *'An estimated one in ten people will have some form of depression, at any one time with it being most common in people aged 25–44 years.'*
>
> WWW.MENTALHEALTH.ORG.UK

Walking and stress

You may be surprised to learn that the main reason many people start a walking routine is not to lose weight or become fit, but to relieve stress. Walking is acknowledged to be a great stress-buster that almost anyone can benefit from. Its ability to relieve stress and tension is down to the endorphins that are released in the brain during exercise. These 'happy hormones' relieve pain and aid relaxation, making you feel calmer, happier and less anxious.

There are various ways in which you can really maximise the stress-busting qualities of walking:

► To get your endorphins flowing at a faster rate, go for a brisk walk.
► To get into a more meditative state, go for a gentle walk and try counting the number of steps you take, focusing on a destination in the distance that you are walking towards or reciting the alphabet in time to your steps. Don't worry if your brain wanders off course (stress is after all what you're trying to relieve!), just acknowledge that it's happened and start again.

> *'...of all exercises, walking is the best'.*
>
> THOMAS JEFFERSON, THIRD PRESIDENT OF THE UNITED STATES
> AND AUTHOR OF THE DECLARATION OF INDEPENDENCE

Walking for the over-50s

It is increasingly important as we age to become and remain active, so that we can delay the onset of health problems common in old age, increase our chance of remaining independent and lead fulfilling, healthy and long lives. Yet with the onset of retirement and children moving away

Hypertension

A certain amount of salt (sodium) is essential in our diet, but too much is a common cause of high blood pressure and can lead to heart disease and other illnesses. Almost all foods contain natural amounts of sodium whereas processed foods are usually laden with added salt. Most of us eat more than the WHO recommended daily amount of salt of 5 grams and should try to reduce our daily intake, particularly if suffering from hypertension. Try these eight tips on how to eat less salt:

1. Look for bread (a major source of sodium) with reduced salt.
2. Buy fresh vegetables rather than canned, which often have salt added.
3. If using produce from a tin, don't cook it in the liquid from the can. Rinse and heat or cook the contents in fresh water.
4. Avoid high salt foods such as salted nuts and crisps.
5. Eat fewer processed foods and ready meals and more fresh produce.
6. Cut back on take-away and fast foods.
7. Buy 'low salt' or 'salt-free' versions of convenience foods.
8. Use herbs and spices such as garlic, oregano, basil and lemon juice to add flavour to meals instead of adding salt to cooking or on the plate.

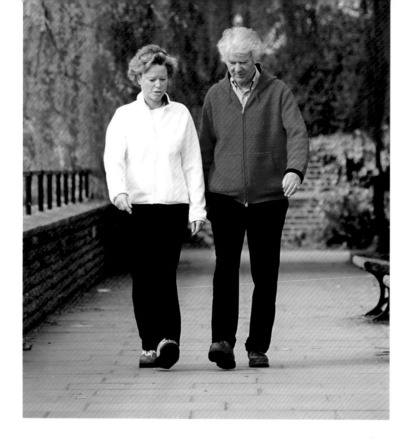

from home, we all too often go from being busy and active to becoming sedentary and sofa-bound. This can lead to a range of conditions from joint stiffness and muscular weakness to osteoporosis, depression, heart disease and stroke.

Walking is the ideal exercise for the over-50s, helping keep bones strong, the heart healthy, confidence high and depression at bay. It is also a great way to meet people – (see Starting your own walking club on page 122). Other medical conditions that can be aided or in some cases prevented by regular walking are:

▶ Strokes.
▶ Alzheimer's disease.
▶ Arthritis.
▶ Asthma.
▶ Lung disease.
▶ High blood pressure/hypertension.
▶ Cancer.

Decide what you want – then go for it

Goals, desires, aims, dreams, targets, wishes: we all have them. What are yours? Maybe it's time for you to start examining these a little more closely, identifying what you want, and starting to progress towards it.

There is a very strong connection between your exercise workout and your life goals in general. Whether your wish is to get a new job, lose weight or become more confident, becoming fit and healthy is an essential first step. As you become more disciplined with what you do with your body and what you put in it, you will inevitably find it easier to take control of other areas of your life, such as your work or family.

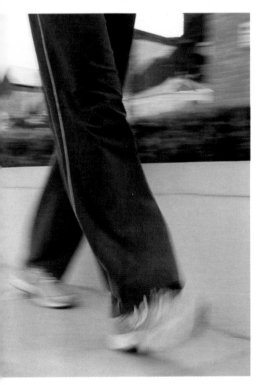

Being specific about what you want is really the crux of getting more from your life. Life whistles by at such a rate that before we realise it we haven't done a fraction of the things we always planned. Don't let regrets pile up. Take control today by deciding what you want, making the positive changes in your life with The WOW! Plan, and ticking those dreams off your list one by one.

Ask any successful person for the secrets of their success and, inevitably, the desire to reach a goal on which they have focused will be right at the top of the list.

Setting SMART goals

Perhaps you have a fair idea of what you would like to achieve. More often than not, we set our sights on something that we would like to accomplish, such as dropping a dress size, getting that promotion or starting our own business, only to fail when we become overwhelmed by what's involved or through lack of persistence.

To give yourself the best chance of sticking with your targets and joining the ranks of those you admire, make sure that your goals are SMART:

Specific – you must have enough information to know exactly what you should be doing when the time comes to do it.
Measurable – you should be able to provide evidence that you have completed your goal.
Attainable – you can reach almost any goal you set yourself if you break it down into manageable steps and timescales. Even the goals that seem out of reach can become possible if you take small steps towards them.
Realistic – only write down goals you intend to follow through. It's better to keep things simple and succeed than to have too many things on your plate and fail. After all, success really does breed success!
Time frame – you must set a time limit for your goal, which could be anything from 1 day to 3 months to 3 years. This is important in helping focus your mind.

Some goals and timescales

Immediate	More energy	To feel brighter and get out of the house
1 month	To be able to walk for 30 mins non-stop	To reduce my medication
3 months	Lose 4kg (9lbs)	Lower blood pressure
6 months	New job	Waist smaller!**
Over 1 year	Stop smoking	Be a size 10!
10 years	Move to a place in the sun	Still be a size 10!

** FOR HELP WITH TAKING BODY MEASUREMENTS, SEE PAGE 47.

If you learn to behave like the person you want to be, whether a successful business executive, slim person, self-made millionaire, good mother or Olympic athlete, you are some of the way there already. Visualise yourself as that person and you will begin to build your self-image and acquire the traits that allow you to reach these goals.

Know what you want, keep focused on what you want and persist until you have achieved it. Write down your goals and place them somewhere visible, like on the fridge door or at your desk, so you can keep referring to them. Look at them every day. If you feel you need help in setting suitable health goals, seek advice from your doctor.

Scales are less important than you think

How often have you stood on the scales in the morning and let the outcome determine how you feel for the rest of day? If you've dropped 2lbs then it feels great, but seeing those numbers increase can really ruin your mood.

Using weight as a measurement of diet, health or fitness success is, however, often erroneous because fluctuations are frequently down to changing water content or heavier muscle tissue. Our bodies are made up of 50–70% water, and how much water we take in or use up on a daily basis can affect what the scales tell us. A weight loss or weight gain could be purely down to being dehydrated or having just drunk some water and nothing at all to do with changing fat content. The weight loss many dieters believe they have achieved is often the result of losing water rather than fat loss, because the person is eating less and depriving themselves of the nutrients they need.

Muscles are heavier than fat (partly because they hold more water), so as you increase your muscle tone with your fitness regime it is possible that this fat loss will be 'cancelled out' on the scales and you'll see no weight change or even weight gain. Do not lose heart. How do those clothes feel? You can drop a size or more without losing weight.

Resist hopping on the scales every morning and concentrate instead on how you look and feel in your clothes as your body shape changes. Why not use your body measurements as a barometer of how well you're doing?

How to fit it in

You are more likely to achieve your daily exercise targets with walking than with any other form of exercise because you can fit them so easily into your daily life. You don't need to travel to a destination to exercise, such as a gym or swimming pool, you don't need to change your clothes and, if pressed for time, you can split your daily target into smaller, more manageable chunks of 10 or 15 minutes throughout the day.

There are various ways in which you can reach your daily walking target:

► Walk to work, school or college rather than taking the car or using public transport.
► Get off the bus or train a stop early and walk the rest of the way.
► Walk instead of using your car for short distances – view it as an opportunity to discover your surroundings, whether you are at work or at home.
► Pop out of the office at lunchtime – you're at work anyway so why not make the most of this 'downtime' and slot your workout easily into the working day. You'll feel brighter in the afternoon and time will fly by – it will be the end of the day before you know it!
► Don't let children stop you from getting outside. Take them with you, and you will all benefit. If they are too young to go very far or really won't be persuaded to join you, perhaps a friend, neighbour or relative could look after them while you do your walk.
► Park your car further away from your destination so you are forced to walk some of the way.
► Arrange to go for a 'walk and chat' with your friend(s) rather than a 'sit and chat' in a local bar or café. You can reward yourselves by going out for a non-alcoholic drink or bite to eat at the end of your walk.

Choosing a route

The beauty of walking is that it can be done in any kind of environment, urban or rural. Riverside and coastal walks, or routes through parks or on public footpaths are obviously wonderful walking environments but there are still plenty of options, even if you don't have parks and rivers nearby. Urban routes, such as along a canal, can be fascinating and walking is often the only way to discover them.

Your local library will have details of interesting and recommended walks in your area. Similarly, your local authority is likely to have produced guides that take you on routes that link historic places and events, interesting buildings and landmarks. These guides generally give you an idea of the time that a given walk will take, the distance covered and convenient start and end points, all of which will help you to plan a really enjoyable outing that suits your level of fitness. If you can vary the terrain that is an advantage, and where there are no hills you can increase the power of your workout by stepping up the pace.

Try to plan a variety of routes for your regular walks. A large-scale map of your home or work area will be extremely useful. The more you vary your route the more you will discover, including new friends where you least expect them, especially if you take a friend magnet commonly known as a 'dog' along with you!

Keeping up your routine while travelling

If your normal routine changes in any way, such as when travelling on business or holiday, it can be difficult to keep up with your health and fitness regime. But with The WOW! Plan it needn't be tough to stay on track. All it takes is a little forward planning and a desire to keep working towards your goals, and you will come back from your trip healthier than ever. Whether you are stressed or over-indulging on the local cuisine on your holiday, walking will help your body cope with the additional strain.

Tips for travelling and walking:

▶ Remember to pack a comfortable pair of trainers to wear for your daily walks while away. If you forget to take your trainers, either use a pair of flat shoes you have with you that are comfortable to walk in or buy another pair of sports shoes. You can then keep that second pair in your suitcase so you'll never be without again.

▶ The concierge or front desk at your hotel should be able to provide you with a jogging map that will offer you a suitable walking route near the hotel. This is a wonderful opportunity to get in a bit of sightseeing on an otherwise work-filled business trip.

▶ Set your alarm call 30 minutes early so you can start the day with a brisk walk to kick-start your metabolism.

▶ If you have early-morning meetings, try to pop out at lunchtime or take a stroll before dinner.

▶ Take the opportunity to explore your surroundings on foot rather than opting for public transport or hiring a car. You'll see far more than you would otherwise and you'll be working out at the same time.

▶ Choose the healthy menu options. Being away from home doesn't mean you can't eat healthily.

Don't let the weather put you off

You can continue your walking plan without letting anyone or anything stop you, including the weather. Don't allow little excuses to creep in to keep you indoors. Recognise them for what they are, excuses, that are testing your determination.

When it's raining or cold, or you just don't feel like going outside, remember what you are working towards. What are you doing this for? Take a moment to focus on what you want to accomplish, and get out there and move towards achieving it. We've all had those evenings when we really didn't fancy going out, but which turned out to be unexpectedly good. The same goes for walking.

If it's cold – stop thinking about it, put on the layers and get going. There's nothing like WOW! walking to warm you up and get your metabolism going. The buzz you feel when you get back is fantastic and you will have worked up a proper appetite too so you can properly enjoy your healthy food.

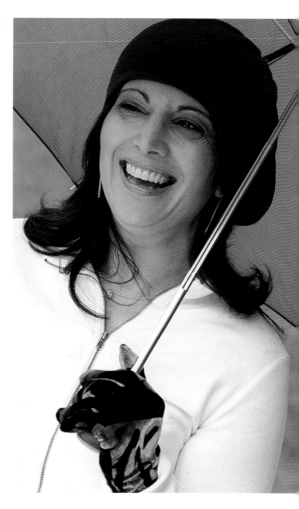

If it's raining don the right gear to keep dry and warm and you will enjoy an immense sense of exhilaration when you get home or back to the office, to know that nothing gets in the way of your workout.

If it's hot – go out in the coolest part of the day or choose a route that's out of the sun and heat, such as a shady riverside or an indoor shopping mall. Wear a hat and cool clothes, take a bottle of water with you to keep hydrated (don't wait until you are thirsty to have a drink – see box opposite) and remember to put on a high SPF sun cream to avoid sunburn.

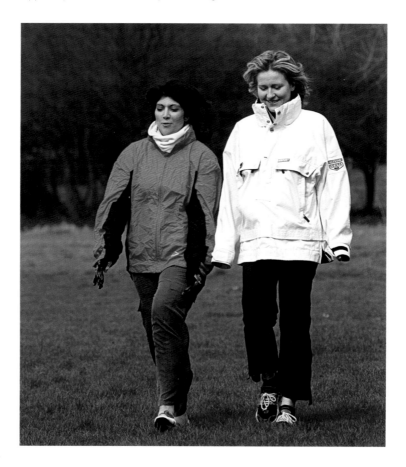

Keeping your water intake up

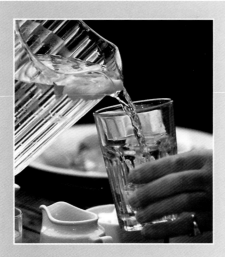

We can last weeks without food, but only days without water. The body is made up of 50–70% water and, because it has no way of storing it, requires fresh supplies every day. Water is so important because it keeps our metabolism working and helps us digest our food.

Most adults lose about 2.5 litres (4.5 pints) per day which they need to replenish by drinking and eating. You will lose more if it is hot or you are pushing yourself particularly hard.

If you keep hydrated throughout the day, you will be less likely to suffer from dehydration during your walk. Here are three tips on getting enough water:

▶ Drink small cups of water throughout the day, ie ½ a cup of water every hour, rather than a large amount in one go.
▶ If you don't like the taste of water, try adding a twist of lemon or lime or some fruit juice.
▶ If you find it difficult to drink enough water, try foods that are good sources of H_2O such as oranges, grapefruit, grapes, watermelon, apples, carrots, tomatoes, tuna, yoghurt, cottage cheese, soups, rice and pasta.

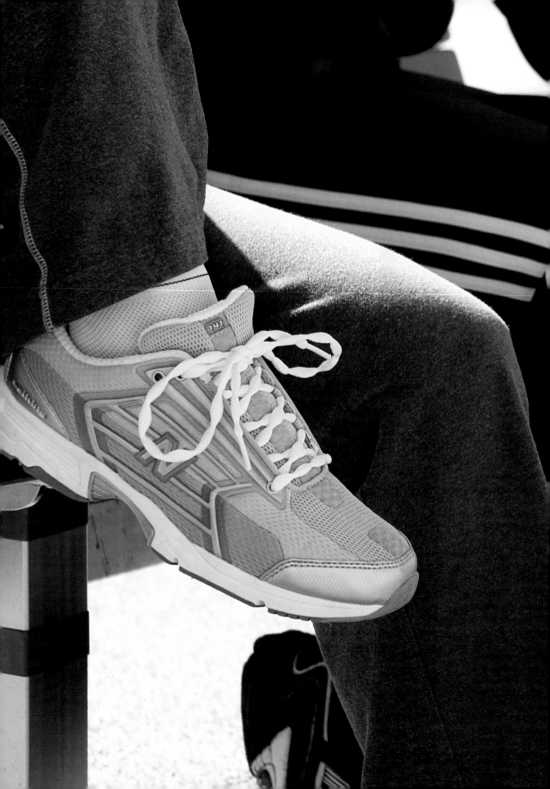

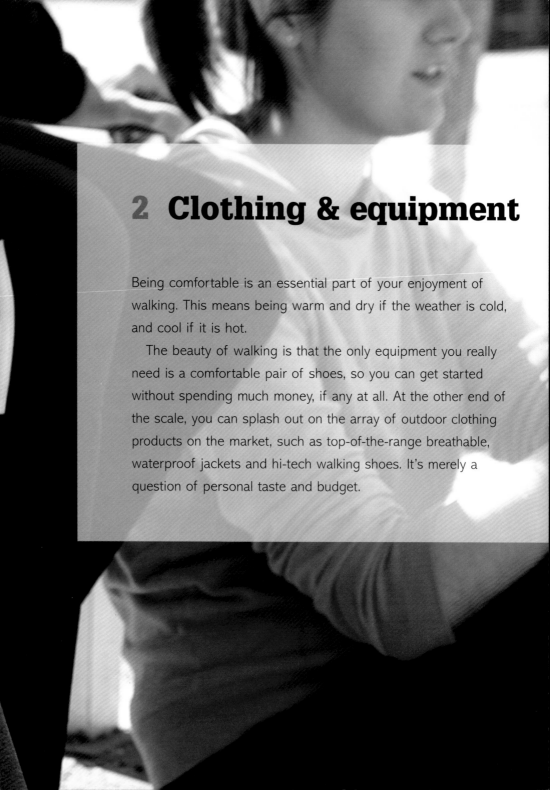

2 Clothing & equipment

Being comfortable is an essential part of your enjoyment of walking. This means being warm and dry if the weather is cold, and cool if it is hot.

The beauty of walking is that the only equipment you really need is a comfortable pair of shoes, so you can get started without spending much money, if any at all. At the other end of the scale, you can splash out on the array of outdoor clothing products on the market, such as top-of-the-range breathable, waterproof jackets and hi-tech walking shoes. It's merely a question of personal taste and budget.

Buying walking shoes

If you decide to invest in a new pair of shoes, there are various options available to you. These include the 'walking' shoes that many manufacturers have brought out to cater to the rapidly growing number of people who choose walking as their primary means of getting fit, running shoes, cross trainers, and hiking shoes or boots. There is no hard-and-fast rule about the type of shoe you should be wearing because what suits you depends on your foot shape, the way you move, the amount, duration and speed you exercise and the surface on which you walk. Walking shoes differ from running shoes in a several different ways:

▶ Walking shoes have a heel that is close to the ground and that curves in, allowing you to roll from heel to toe as you walk. Running shoes have a thicker, higher heel that often flares out. When walking, this can cause your foot to slap down rather than roll (and lead to sore shins – see page 39).
▶ Walking shoes have a stiffer sole which makes them more stable but less flexible than a running shoe.
▶ The uppers of walking shoes are often made from leather or similar-looking synthetic material.
▶ A good walking shoe will have a firm heel and rear foot cushioning, although a walking shoe will never provide as much cushioning as a running shoe.

As your fitness levels increase and you are walking faster, for longer, you may want to swap your walking shoe for a running shoe. The extra cushioning in a running shoe can protect you against the increased injury risk associated with exercising for long periods of time on roads or other hard surfaces.

Cross trainers can be an economical option, allowing you to buy one pair of shoes that perform a variety of activities. They are functional and versatile, providing suitable cushioning and support for different types of exercise. They generally have wider, more stable soles than running shoes to provide lateral movement support, but are similar to walking shoes in that they are heavier and less flexible than your average running shoe.

Hiking shoes or boots are designed to protect your feet and ankles from rugged terrain. A good hiking boot should be waterproof, with a treaded, high-grip outsole and a high cut to prevent ankle sprains. These shoes are not suitable for urban or fitness walking on level ground because their rigidity does not allow your foot sufficient movement.

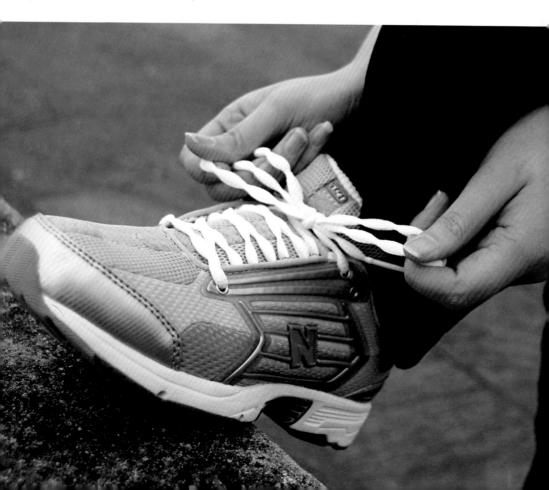

A few things to remember when buying shoes:

- ► Choose shoes by how they feel on your feet, not just by the size marked. Sizes vary by style, brand and country of manufacture.
- ► Make sure you can wiggle your toes freely in the front of the shoe, but don't buy them so loose that your feet slide around.
- ► Try on shoes with socks or any special inserts you normally wear.
- ► Allow a gap the size of the width of your index finger between the tip of your longest toe and the front of the shoe.
- ► Make sure your heels don't slip around in the shoes. Test them out by walking around the store before you buy.
- ► Don't expect shoes to stretch.
- ► Buy shoes at the end of the day. The longer you are on your feet, the more they swell.
- ► Alternate between two pairs of shoes and you'll save money in the long run. 'Resting' your shoes every other day delays their deterioration and allows them to bounce back.
- ► Change your shoes every 650–7000 km (400–600 miles)!

Adjusting your shoe to your foot movements

Pronation refers to the inward roll of the foot during normal walking motion and occurs as the outer edge of the heel strikes the ground and the foot rolls inward and flattens out. **Supination** is the opposite of pronation and refers to the outward roll of the foot during normal walking motion.

If you have a tendency to either excessive pronation or supination you may suffer pains and sprains in the foot, ankle, knees, hips and back. Ask your retailer for advice – suitable shoes and/or inserts could help balance out the problem.

Preventing injuries

Walking is a low-impact activity which carries little risk of injury, but most walkers experience muscle soreness, shin splints or blisters at some point. Minimise your chances of these by preparing properly and knowing how to treat any problems quickly should they arise.

Muscle soreness

Some level of mild, general muscle soreness is to be expected when you start exercising for the first time after a period of inactivity. If this happens, allow your body the rest that it needs to recuperate and repair the muscles that have been used. As you become fitter and leaner and your muscles become stronger, you will be able to exercise for longer and harder without muscle soreness. Take it slowly at first, gradually increasing the amount you exercise and the effort you put in. Stretching is the key so make sure you warm up and cool down properly (see page 73). It is also important to adopt correct posture and walking technique (page 76–77) so that you do not put undue strain on your back. Walk tall and do not overstretch by reaching your foot too far out in front of your body – take shorter strides out front while extending your stride at the back.

If you experience a sharp pain or a burning sensation, stop immediately and rest the area. Ice the painful spot, keep it compressed and keep it elevated, preferably above your heart. If you think you might have caused some damage, take it easy for a day or two, stop exercising and see if the pain subsides. If the pain persists, seek advice from a medical professional.

Shin splints

Shin soreness or shin splints are quite common, particularly when people start exercising by doing too much too soon. You can prevent shin pain by wearing a well-fitted shoe (a running shoe is probably best) which provides cushioning under your heel, as well as walking on soft surfaces such as grass rather than stomping on hard pavements or tracks.

Blisters

You've probably suffered from a blister at some time in your life. The secret of blister prevention is to keep your feet dry. To prevent blisters:

- ► Wear socks made from a 'wicking' fabric such as CoolMax(c) or polypropylene thats draw moisture away from your feet.
- ► Avoid cotton socks.
- ► Change into dry socks as soon as possible in the event of your feet becoming wet.
- ► Spray your feet with antiperspirant if excessive moisture continues to be a problem.
- ► Cover a hot spot with a blister pad, available from pharmacies and many supermarkets, to keep it protected and prevent it from turning into a full-blown blister.

If a blister occurs, swab the area with rubbing alcohol, drain it by pricking the blister close to the edge with a sterilised needle (do not rub or remove the skin covering the blister), apply some antiseptic and then cover the area with bandage or a gauze. Change the dressing daily. The best tip is to carry some blister pads with you on your walks so that you can apply them to any hot spots before they have a chance to develop further.

To prevent any of these potential problems hindering your enjoyment of walking, visit a good sports store and be fitted for the correct athletic shoes for your feet and the amount and type of exercise you will be doing.

Keeping warm

The best and most versatile way to keep warm is to wear thin layers of clothing. Air is trapped between the layers, which keep you warm. When you become hot, you can peel off a layer or two to regulate your body temperature closely.

It is important to keep your extremities covered up in cold weather – we lose up to 75% of our body heat through our heads. To fight the cold:

▶ Wear a hat to prevent warm air from escaping. Hats that cover your ears may also be helpful preventing earache in cold winds.
▶ Keep your neck warm by covering it completely with a scarf or high-necked top.
▶ Wear gloves (mittens are best as they allow the warm air to circulate) to protect your hands.

The best materials to wear next to your skin are natural fibres such as silk, cotton and wool, with outer layers in fleece, which works because it is both warm and windproof.

NB If you go out in the dark during short winter days, be sure to wear bright colours or something reflective so that motorists and cyclists can see you clearly.

Keeping dry

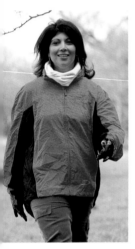

On a hot day, a rainstorm might be quite pleasant to cool you off. But when it's cold, the last thing you want is to become wet.

When buying outer clothing, check whether the materials used are waterproof or showerproof, breathable and/or windproof. Examples of the many types of breathable, waterproof materials on the market include Isotex(c), Indra(c), Gore-Tex(c), Sympatex(c) and Scantex(c). Prices vary greatly according to the brand but there is nothing to choose between them in quality – you can spend as little or as much as you like.

Lightweight, non-breathable kagoul-type tops, which are low cost, might be suitable when walking in the autumn and spring months in mild climates. In wilder and wetter winter months, however, go for heavier duty, breathable jackets. If you are walking in the city, you are naturally more protected from the elements than when walking out in exposed, open countryside or coastal areas. Make sure you choose the most robust clothing in exposed environments.

Tips for buying waterproof clothing:

► Choose breathable materials that draw moisture away from your skin as you become hot, so reducing the 'clammy' feeling you can experience with non-breathable material such as PVC.

► Look for hoods with peaks as these keep rain away from your face. Check for adjustable cords that allow you to tighten the hood around your face in windy weather.

► Go for versatile 2-in-1 jackets which include an inner detachable fleece layer for warmth. You can wear the inner layer on its own for warmth on cold, dry days, the outer waterproof shell on warm but wet days and both together when it's freezing and wet!

► Buy waterproof trousers that have long zips in the legs so they are easy to pull on and take off over trousers and boots.

Keeping cool

On hot days, keeping up your water intake and making sure that you wear clothes which reduce the impact of heat and sun are your most important considerations.

Tips for keeping cool:

▶ Wear a hat to shade yourself from the sun.

▶ Keep hydrated – take water with you and drink regularly. Don't wait until you are thirsty because by that time you are already dehydrated.

▶ Wear sunglasses to protect your eyes from the sun's harmful ultraviolet rays. Sunglasses can also make you feel cooler by giving you the impression that you are walking in the shade.

▶ Wear clothing that is designed to draw moisture away from your skin. Examples of these hi-tech fabrics are CoolMax(c) and DriFit(c). Loose-fitting and light-coloured clothing is best.

▶ Walk during the coolest part of the day, either early morning or early evening. If it is still too hot, consider walking inside, such as in a shopping arcade.

▶ Don't overdo it. If you feel yourself overheating, always stop and rest for a while.

For your back pack

As well as your bottle of water, take an energy snack, some plasters in case of blisters and your mobile phone in case of emergency.

Gadgets – measuring your progress

Now that you've decided what you're doing and why, let's move on to how you're going to monitor your progress.

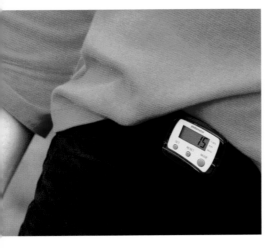

Pedometers/stepometers

These are fantastic, inexpensive little gadgets which have been much talked about recently with the government-endorsed initiative to walk 10,000 steps per day. They measure the number of steps you take and, depending on the model you buy, can also measure distance walked and calories burned. Some require that you calibrate them by inputting your weight and step length while others work on a pre-determined average stride length.

Pedometers are useful in motivating you to exercise towards a specific goal. To get as accurate a reading as possible, attach the device to the front of your waistband, directly above the knee. Bear in mind that the distance walked and calories burned will be underestimated if you work especially hard during your walking session, such as by walking uphill or particularly briskly, because the pedometer is not calibrated to measure intensity of effort.

If you complete the 10,000 steps per day now recommended by governments and health professionals, you will have:

- ▶ Burned about 300–400 calories per day, depending on your walking speed and body size.
- ▶ Walked about 8 km (5 miles);
- ▶ Burned 2,000–3,500 extra calories per week.

Heart Rate Monitors (HRMs)

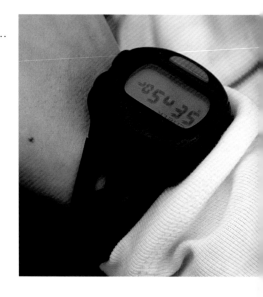

Owning a Heart Rate Monitor is like having your very own personal trainer. HRMs measure your heart rate but can offer a wide range of additional functions as well, depending on the model. The most useful function to look out for when purchasing an HRM is the ability to exercise within a set target zone. This allows you to be more specific about how hard or gently you wish to exercise. If your heart rate falls below the lower limit or rises above the higher limit, the monitor will beep to warn you to either work harder or slow down to get back into the target zone.

When we exercise, we burn both fat and carbohydrate. In order to maximise our ability to burn fat rather than carbohydrate, we must exercise at low to moderate intensity levels. While you burn more calories the harder you exercise, the level at which you burn the highest level of fat in relation to carbohydrate is relatively low, namely between 60% and 75% of your maximum heart rate. This is commonly known as the 'Fat Burning Zone'. Walking, and in particular walking with the WOW! techniques is therefore an ideal way of optimising your fat-burning potential.

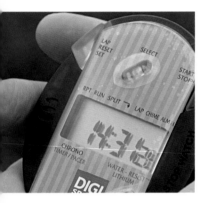

Pacer stopwatch

This gadget will keep you walking at a set rate. This is useful as the mental relaxation which develops when you are walking can cause you to slow down. Pacer stopwatches not only give you an accurate record of the duration of your exercise, but can be set to beep at a regular pace. This is a great help in enabling you to maintain the same pace without having to think about it, so that you can enjoy the sights and sounds during your walk.

Working out your Fat Burning Zone

To find your Fat Burning Zone, you must first work out your maximum heart rate. An easy way to do this is to subtract your age from 220. **NB** if you are on high blood pressure medication, your maximum heart rate may be lower. Check with your doctor.

Example – a 35-year-old man or woman
▶ 220 minus 35 gives a MHR of 185
▶ 60% of the MHR gives the lower 'Fat Burning' limit:
  60/100 x 185 = 111
▶ 75% of the MHR gives the upper 'Fat Burning' limit:
  75/100 x 185 = 139
So, for a person of 35 to maximise their potential to burn fat, they should keep their heart rate between 111 and 139 beats per minute – their Fat Burning Zone.

Please note that this is a general guide and does not take into consideration other factors, such as when you are feeling unwell. However, the most sophisticated HRMs will give you accurate limits adjusted to take account of your current state of health into account.

Body measurements

Measuring your progress on a healthy lifestyle programme is an important motivator to keep you focused on your goals. You'll be feeling better as soon as you start The WOW! Plan, but it's always good to see those numbers changing!

There are various ways in which you can monitor your measurements on a regular basis:

BMI (Body Mass Index)

Inch-loss is more important than weight loss, for all the reasons previously discussed. However, it can be helpful to measure your Body Mass Index (BMI) at the outset, particularly if you are overweight, because this will give you a yardstick by which to improve. The BMI is largely accepted as the international standard in measuring someone's weight in relation to their height.

Do bear in mind that the BMI is a very general measure and does not differentiate between fat, muscle and bone weight. For example, a body builder with 8% body fat will probably have a BMI in the 'obese' category because his muscles are so heavy.

Taking your body measurements

You will start to realise that your body has shrunk when you can get into your clothes more easily, but it is useful to take regular body measurements to reinforce how well you're doing.

All you need is a tape measure: ideally take your waist, hip and thigh measurements every 8 to 10 weeks. When measuring, use a full-length mirror to ensure the tape is level all the way around.

Measuring your BMI

To calculate your BMI, you need to know your weight and height.

Stage 1 Work out your height in metres and square the figure (see the conversion table below).

Imperial	Metric (cm)	Imperial	Metric (cm)
4'8"	142	5'6"	167.5
4'9"	144.5	5'7"	170
4'10"	147	5'8"	172.5
4'11"	150	5'9"	175
5'	152.5	5'10"	177.5
5'1"	155	5'11"	180
5'2"	157.5	6'	183
5'3"	160	6'1"	185.5
5'4"	162.5	6'2"	188
5'5"	165	6'3"	190.5

Stage 2 Measure your weight in kilograms (to convert pounds to kilograms multiply by 0.45).

Stage 3 Divide your weight (stage 2) by your height squared (stage 1) to get your BMI.

Example A person is 5'7" tall and weights 70kg:

▶ 5'7"/1.7m x 1.7 = 2.89m

▶ 70 ÷ 2.89 = 24.2

▶ BMI = 24.2

With a BMI of 24.2, this individual falls within the normal weight category of 18.5–25.

18.5 underweight   **18.5–25** normal weigh   **25–30** overweight   **30** obese

- Waist – measure where your body is narrowest (about 1 inch above your navel). If your waist does not go in, measure around your navel.
- Hips – measure at your widest point.
- Thighs – measure your right thigh at the widest point.

Measuring your resting heart rate

The average resting heart rate is between 60 and 80 beats per minute. As a general rule, the lower your resting heart rate, the fitter you are and vice versa.

- **To measure the pulse at your wrist** Place your index and middle finger over the underside of the opposite wrist, below the base of the thumb. Press firmly with flat fingers until you feel the pulse.
- **To measure the pulse on your neck** Place the index and middle finger just to the side of the Adam's apple, in the soft hollow area. Press firmly until the pulse is located.
- **Once you find the pulse** Count the beats for 15 seconds and multiply by 4. This will give the beats per minute.

Music

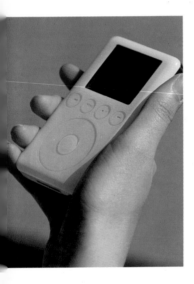

Listening to music while you walk is a great way to help the time and miles fly by.

You'll get most out of it if you make up your own compilation, using slower tracks at the start and end of your walking session for the warm-up and cool-down periods, and higher tempo tracks in between to help you keep your pace up during the main workout. It has been shown that music which has more beats per minute (bpm) leads to a higher heart rate – not surprisingly, faster music really does make you go faster and work harder.

Your walking range is about 110 bpm to 150 bpm (100 bpm being slow walking, 130 bpm brisk walking and 150 bpm fast walking). Roughly, these work out to the following speeds:

- ▶ 110 bpm = 5 km/h (3 mph)
- ▶ 120 bpm = 5.6 km/h (3.5 mph)
- ▶ 130 bpm = 6.4 km/h (4 mph)
- ▶ 140 bpm = 7.2 km/h (4.5 mph)
- ▶ 150 bpm = 8 km/h (5 mph)

Some walking CDs or cassettes are music only while others include instruction and motivation voiceovers throughout. Go to www.workoutwalking.com to link to various sites that sell walking CDs.

Safety first

Make sure you stay safe when out and about. Wearing a personal stereo can put you at risk of being knocked over by a bike or make you easy prey snatchers, so be extra vigilant when listening to music. Choose the area you walk in carefully, opting for light, open and populated areas rather than dark and quiet places and remove or turn off your portable music player when crossing a road.

It's got a good beat...

To give you an idea, here's a list of well-known songs and their approximate bpm:

80 bpm	Beautiful	Christina Aguilera
95 bpm	Here I Go Again	Whitesnake
110 bpm	I Have a Dream	Abba
	If I Could Turn Back Time	Cher
115 bpm	Hot in the City	Billy Idol
120 bpm	Addicted to Love	Robert Palmer
	California Girls	The Beach Boys
	Respect	Aretha Franklin
125 bpm	Escape	Enrique Iglesias
	Don't Stop Moving	S Club 7
130 bpm	Can You Feel It?	The Jacksons
	Get Back	The Beatles
	Rocks	Primal Scream
140 bpm	It's Raining Men	The Weather Girls
	A Hard Day's Night	The Beatles
150 bpm	Waterloo	Abba
180 bpm	Dead Ringer for Love	Meat Loaf

Work out the BPMs of your favourite tracks To do this, tap your foot in time to the music and count the number of taps over a 60-second period. Alternatively, count for a period of 15 seconds and multiply by 4 to work out the beats per minute.

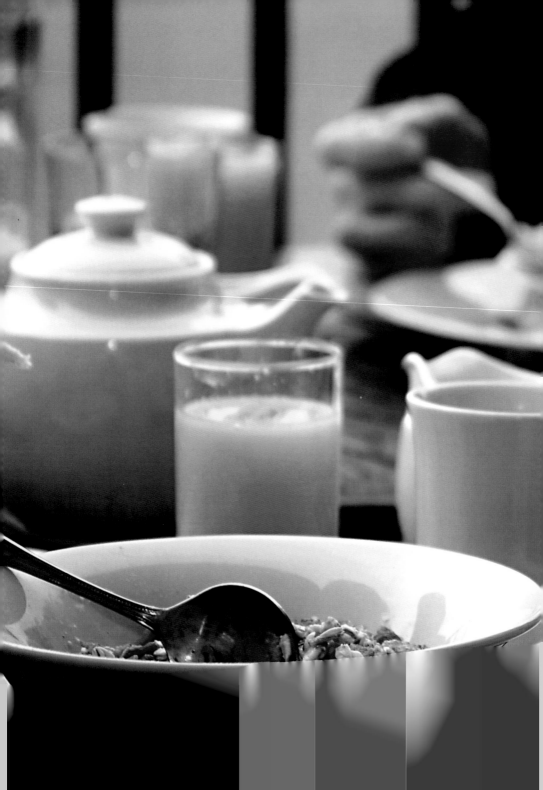

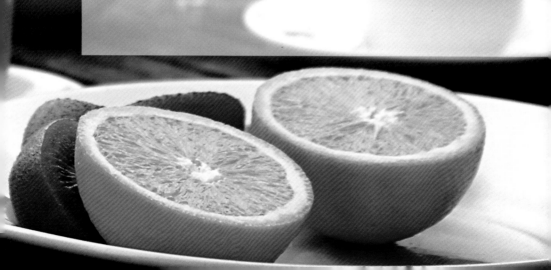

3 Eating & exercise

Walking Fit is a book about how to get fit and healthy by walking. It is not a book about dieting. However, food and exercise go together, so before you move on to The Workout Walking (WOW!) Plan you need to make sure you know how to prepare for your new active life and get more energy and drive from the food you eat. After all, you are what you eat! If you eat predominantly fatty, processed foods, you will be overweight, unfocused and lacking in energy. If you choose a tasty balance of all the food groups, prepared in a healthy way, you will be lean and bursting with vitality. Which would you prefer?

A little of everything does you good

In the Western world, dieting has become inextricably linked to eating. Whether we're talking about it, eating it or buying it, when it comes to food it seems that we're almost solely concerned with whether or not it will help us lose or gain weight. And it's easy to see why.

Today's media-driven world is obsessed with how we look, holding up stick-thin celebrities as the ultimate symbols of success and beauty. This is where the problem lies: beautiful often means thin. If we could just become as thin as our role models, we think, wouldn't we be as successful and happy as they seem to be?

Energy and where it comes from

Calories provide our bodies with the energy they need to function properly. A calorie is a unit of energy that comes from the food that we eat. If you are looking to lose or maintain weight, the solution is quite simple:

If you consume (eat) more calories than you expend (by physical activity), they will be stored as fat and you will put on weight. If you consume fewer calories than you burn, by eating less and/or exercising more, you will lose weight. If you burn the same number of calories as you consume, your weight will stay the same.

Carbohydrates and proteins both provide 4 calories per gram, whereas fats provide more than twice that, at 9 calories per gram. Fat is therefore more densely packed with energy, and it is for this reason that it is advisable to limit the amount of fat you eat.

Any calories we don't use, we wear!

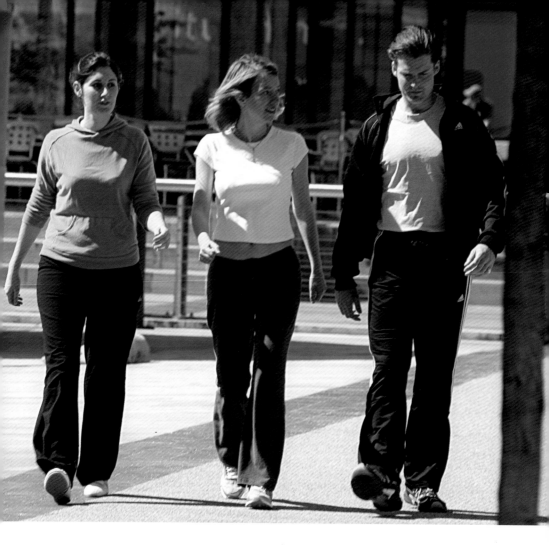

So we go on a diet. And we deprive ourselves of sufficient quantities of the three macronutrients – carbohydrates, proteins and fats – not to mention other essential vitamins and minerals contained in a variety of foods. This not only fails to deliver long-term weight loss but can be downright dangerous. Our bodies require a balance of all the food groups and will suffer if denied any one of them.

The only solution to long-term weight management is one that also leads to good health. Quite simply, it is a combination of eating a varied diet of nutritious food and exercising to burn off any excess calories before they can turn to fat.

The Health Bank

We have a natural tendency to focus more attention on the good things that we do for our health than the bad things. If we choose a salad rather than a fast-food burger for lunch, go to the gym before work or eat a piece of fruit instead of a chocolate bar, we feel good that we have done something positive for our health.

Now take a moment to think about some of the things that you do that may have a negative impact on your health. What about the coffee you had for breakfast, the beer at lunchtime or the car you used to go to work instead of walking? If you're anything like me, you tend to gloss over these, choosing to concentrate on the good stuff instead.

Compare this to how we deal with our bank accounts. While it's true that some of us have a mental block when it comes to money, generally we are much more aware of what goes both in and out of our bank account. Most of us try not to spend more than we have as the results can be painful.

With our health it is a different story. The human body can put up with an enormous amount of abuse before it shows signs of ill health. But the damage is still being done. Payback time will come – and it could be sooner and more serious than you expect.

With The WOW! Plan you'll learn to start thinking of your health in the same way as you do your bank account. Think about the debits, the negative things that you do to your body as well as the credits, the positive things that boost your 'health balance'. Write down your credits and debits and become conscious of how you can reduce your debits and increase your credits. Boost your health bank by:

▶ Walking to work or to the local shop instead of taking the car or using public transport.
▶ Limiting yourself to one alcoholic drink a day or cutting out alcohol completely during the week and just having a couple at the weekend.
▶ Treating yourself to comfort food once a week on a Friday.

What is the link between food and exercise?

When we exercise, our muscles require fuel to move our bodies. This fuel is the energy we get from our food. If we become hungry, our muscles can run out of energy, and we become weak, tired and unable to get the most out of our workout. On the other hand, being too full of food before exercising can cause problems because blood is being diverted to our stomachs to digest our food rather than to our muscles to keep them functioning. It is therefore essential that we eat enough food, of the right type and at the right time, so that we remain able to function properly.

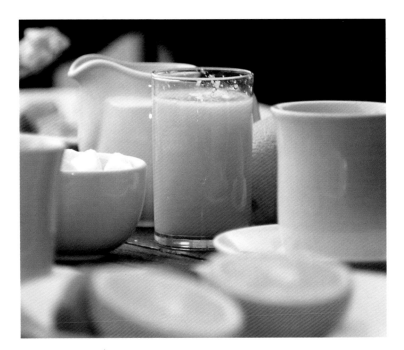

When to eat

With The WOW! Plan, you can eat up to 1 hour before exercising. This should be a healthy, energy-giving snack rather than a full-blown meal, allowing you time to digest it before calling on your energy reserves for exercise. You should also eat 45 minutes to 1 hour after exercising to allow your body to replenish and repair itself. If you decide to fit your daily session in first thing in the morning, you can do so before breakfast (drink a small cup of water before you leave to remain hydrated); there should be enough stored energy left in your body from your meal the night before, and you can boost your metabolism on your return with a nutritious breakfast.

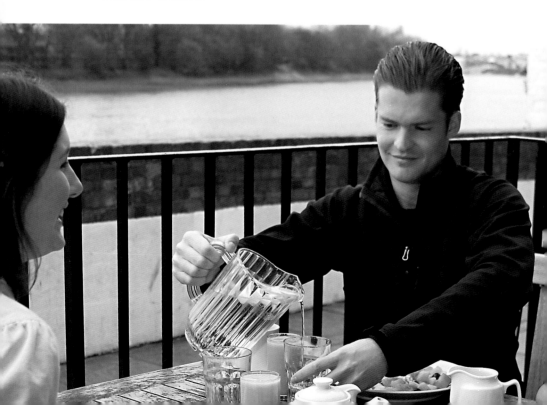

Eating sugar at the wrong time
can be bad when exercising...

Sugar is a simple carbohydrate which when eaten causes our blood glucose levels to rise rapidly. This triggers our pancreas to produce insulin to return our glucose levels to normal. The problem arises when a sudden peak stimulates the pancreas to produce too much insulin, leading to low blood sugar levels up to 5 hours after the sugar has been eaten. This can cause tiredness, irritability and the desire for yet more sweet food (which often lacks nutrients) – it's easy to see how this can lead to see-saw eating. By eating more complex carbohydrates that take longer to be broken down in the digestive system (in addition to being more nutritious), you will encourage a gradual release of energy and avoid the stress and strain on the body that comes from having to redress unhealthy sugar imbalances. This will help you exercise to your full potential.

What to eat around exercise

This is where people can differ, so the best thing is to experiment with various foods to see what suits you best.

Before exercising, you should eat a light, balanced snack of complex carbohydrate, protein and a small amount of fat. Carbohydrates are the most easily digested and primary source of energy for the body, so will boost your energy during exercise as well as replenishing energy stores when you get back. Try to eat a slow-burning complex carbohydrate, such as brown bread or brown rice, before you exercise in order to keep your blood sugar levels even and to allow steady energy release over the period that you exercise. On your return, if you are tired after a hard workout, eat a simple carbohydrate such as a banana to quickly restore your blood sugar levels before they dip too low. Protein is particularly helpful in repairing your muscles after they have been used.

Quick guide to daily eating for best performance

To really get the most out of your walks, it is important that you not only eat properly around your exercise sessions, but that your general diet is balanced and nutritious.

As mentioned earlier, a well-balanced approach to living means having a bit of everything in your diet. For optimum health and energy your daily diet should consist of approximately:

60% carbohydrate This is the main source of energy for your body and the primary fuel for your brain.

▶ **Make sure the majority of this 60% is from complex carbohydrates ('starches' or polysaccharides).** These are made up of many sugar units linked together to form 'complex' molecules, which take longer for your body to digest. The result is that you stay full for longer and don't suffer erratic shifts in energy levels. Complex carbohydrates also provide vitamins and minerals. Examples are vegetables, whole grains, seeds and beans.

▶ **Limit the amount of simple carbohydrates you eat.** Simple carbohydrates (also called sugars, monosaccharides, disaccharides or oligosaccharides) are made up of between one and three units of sugar linked together. They are quickly and easily digested into the bloodstream. The sudden surge of energy they produce can be destabilising for your body, leading to peaks and troughs in your energy levels. Examples of simple carbohydrates include honey, jams, sweets, soft drinks, sugar, white rice, white bread, white pasta and other white flour products. An exception to this is fruit. Although fruits are simple carbohydrates and high in natural sugar, they provide a range of vitamins and should be an important part of your diet.

Fruit and vegetables will
help you reach your max!

Numerous studies have shown that a high intake of fruit and vegetables may lower an individual's risk of getting illnesses such as heart disease and certain cancers. They provide a wide range of vitamins and minerals that you need to function properly. Governments and healthcare professionals recommend that you eat at least five portions of fruit and vegetables every day (not including potatoes). While fresh is best, tinned, frozen, cooked, juiced or dried portions also count. Here's a suggestion from the UK Food Standards Agency for your five daily portions:

1 Glass of pink grapefruit juice for breakfast (1 portion) (shop-bought juice only counts as 1 portion, no matter how much you drink. Bear in mind that fruit juice contains a large amount of natural sugar).
2 Small pack of dried apricots for mid-morning snack, instead of that chocolate bar or bag of crisps (1 portion).
3 Side salad with lunch (1 portion).
4 Sugar snap peas and asparagus, served with main meal (1 portion).
5 Strawberries as dessert (1 portion).

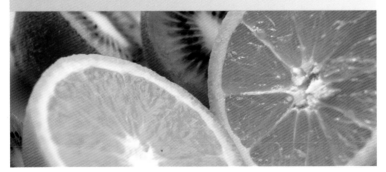

15–30% fats Fats keep us warm, help protect our organs and help move nutrients around the body.

The best types of fats to eat are:

▶ **Monounsaturated** the healthiest type of fat because they reduce the amount of LDL (bad cholesterol – see page 62) in our body. They are found in olive, rapeseed, canola and sesame seed oils, avocados, nuts and seeds.

▶ **Polyunsaturated** found in most vegetable oils such as corn, safflower, sunflower and soybean oils. (These should not be used to fry food, as they turn into Trans Fatty Acids – see below.)

▶ **Essential Fatty Acids** made up of Omega 6 Fatty Acids (found in unrefined safflower, corn, sesame and sunflower oils) and Omega 3 Fatty Acids (found in oily fish, linseed/flax, hemp and soybean oils, pumpkin seeds, walnuts, dark green vegetables).

▶ **Avoid saturated fats where possible** These are found in animal foods (meat, cheese, eggs, dairy) and some oils like palm kernel oil and Trans-Fatty Acids which are created when unsaturated fats are 'cooked' (hydrogenated) and turned into saturated fats. TFAs are found mainly in margarines and vegetable fat, and are particularly unhealthy because they are thought to reduce 'good' cholesterol (HDL) while increasing 'bad' cholesterol (LDL). Consumed in excess, these fats can cause weight gain and may lead to a narrowing of the arteries which can cause heart disease.

10–15% protein Much of the body, such as brain cells, muscles, skin, hair and nails, is made up of protein. Protein is essential because it breaks down to amino acids which repair and maintain the body. Sources of protein include animal products like meat, poultry and fish, eggs and dairy products and plants such as seeds, nuts, beans, lentils and soy products as well as grains, especially wheat. There are about 20 amino acids, which can be split into two groups: those that can be made by the body (non-essential amino acids) and those that cannot be made by the body and so must be taken in by food (essential amino acids).

Power up breakfast time!

Whether you've gone out first thing to fit your walk into your day or you're going out later on, give yourself the chance to start the day the right way by eating a nutritious breakfast. Breakfast is the most important meal of the day yet tends to be the one most often skipped.

Breakfast is important because by feeding the brain, it helps you perform better throughout the day. Eating breakfast also boosts your body's metabolic rate which means that you burn calories at a greater rate all through the day than you would if breakfast had been skipped. It is therefore easier to control your weight if you have a healthy breakfast every morning.

Don't rely on coffee and sugary foods to set you up for your action-packed day. Choose foods that feed your brain and provide slow-releasing energy to take you through to lunchtime, such as those foods that are high in fibre and protein and low in fat. Remember, the aim each and every day is to keep your blood sugar levels as even as possible so as to avoid the peaks and troughs that affect energy levels, moods and performance. That means slow-burning (complex) carbohydrates, protein and a small amount of fat (preferably unsaturated).

Breakfast ideas

▶ **Yoghurt** Try natural, live, low-fat yoghurt with no added sugar rather than sugary fruit yoghurts. Live yoghurt provides 'friendly' bacteria that aid your digestive system. To make it more nutritious, add uncooked porridge oats (high in fibre), chopped nuts or seeds (high in protein and beneficial fats), sliced or chopped fruit (fresh or dried) and/or powdered cinnamon (the spice has been shown to benefit those with type 2 diabetes, reduce LDL cholesterol, aid digestion and stimulate circulation).

▶ **Fresh fruit** Start the day by eating ½ a grapefruit, a banana or an orange. This alone won't be enough to keep you going for very long, so combine it with something like yoghurt or cereal (preferably sugar-free and low salt) to provide a more satisfying meal.

▶ **Porridge** Widely acknowledged to reduce bad cholesterol. Cook oats in milk or water (or a mixture of both). Add nuts, seeds, fresh or dried fruit (try to avoid adding sugar or salt) for a delicious, warming start to the day. For a change, try using millet or rice flakes instead of oats. These alternatives are available at health food stores and, increasingly, in supermarkets.

▶ **Toast** Use brown rather than white bread. Don't just stick to the old favourite spreads like marmalade, jam (jelly) or yeast spreads (Marmite/Vegemite). Instead experiment with toppings that are more filling, such as cheese and tomato, tuna or a poached egg. Use butter or margarine containing no hydrogenated fat (check the label).

▶ **Traditional fry-up** There's nothing wrong with the full English breakfast once in a while, but make this a healthier option by grilling the sausages and bacon, toasting the bread and poaching the eggs rather than frying everything in fat.

▶ **Cereal** Pick non-sweetened varieties such as muesli with no added sugar, or wheat or bran flakes. Beware, most breakfast cereals are laden with sugar, salt and additives. Add fruit and/or nuts for a more wholesome breakfast and to add sweetness.

▶ **Milk** Skimmed or semi-skimmed is healthier than full fat because it contains less saturated fat. For variety, try soya, rice or oat milk.

▶ **Juice** Make sure that this is 100% juice. Avoid products labelled 'juice drink' because they contain a lot of sugar and not a lot of fruit. Try flavours other than orange, such as apple, grapefruit, prune or cranberry.

▶ **Water** The only true thirst quencher. Try to substitute your morning dose of coffee for herbal tea or hot water, lemon and grated fresh ginger. Or just a mineral water. Your body and skin will thank you for it.

▶ **Sugar** Sugar contains nothing but empty calories so try to sweeten your food with fresh or dried fruit or honey instead.

Daytime 'fuelling' tips

Do you ever get that sleepy feeling in the afternoon following lunch, when all you really want to do is lie down for a power nap? This is largely due to a natural phenomenon, when our body rhythms slow down our metabolism between about 2pm and 4pm, making us feel tired. So it's important to boost your energy levels in the middle of the day as the energy from your breakfast wears off and so avoid as far as is possible that dreaded drowsy feeling.

Lunchtime

▶ If you choose to go walking in your lunch break, take a light snack (see Snack Time below) about 1 hour before you go out, followed by another snack when you return, rather than one bigger meal in the middle of the day. This will ensure that you have sufficient energy both during and after your workout, without suffering dips in your blood sugar levels.

▶ Try to eat less at lunch and have a snack ready for when your energy is at its lowest in the middle of the afternoon. When we eat, blood and oxygen are sent to our stomachs to break down the food that we've eaten and get the digestive process under way. The more we eat, the more energy is required to digest it, leaving our brains with less 'fuel' to keep us alert, productive and awake. Eat less at lunchtime, therefore, and your brain will be left with more energy to keep you on form through the afternoon.

▶ Avoid fatty, fried foods at lunchtime. They are hard to digest and channel much of the body's blood and oxygen away from the brain and into the digestive system.

▶ Try to avoid eating simple carbohydrates, such as sugar, sweets and white bread or pasta. These cause a sharp peak and then a rapid fall in blood sugar, leading to low energy and afternoon sleepiness.

▶ Adopt a balanced approach to lunch, with a mixture of complex carbohydrates, some protein and a small amount of fat. For example, a crunchy salad with protein such as hard-boiled egg, chicken or tuna and oil dressing, a houmous and salad pitta bread (preferably brown) or chicken and sweetcorn soup with buttered bread.

Snack time

If you feel your energy dropping between your main meals, avoid the temptation to reach for a sweet or salty snack, and try some of these delicious healthy alternatives:

Before and after exercising
▶ Yoghurt with oats, nuts and honey.
▶ Vegetarian omelette with a slice of toast (preferably wholemeal).
▶ Chicken and brown rice salad.
▶ Tuna or salmon sandwich.
▶ Boiled egg and a piece of toast.
▶ Bacon sandwich.
▶ Vegetable sticks dipped in houmous, guacamole or tzatziki.
▶ Sprouted beans, nuts, seeds and grains.

Post-exercise quick fixes if your energy has dipped – do NOT eat these before exercising because they will cause your energy levels to dip.
▶ Fresh fruit eg banana.
▶ Dried fruit.
▶ Honey on toast.
▶ Jacket potato with sweetcorn or low-fat filling.
▶ Cereal bar.
▶ Low-fat cream cheese spread on a rice cake, corn cake or Ryvita.

Shopping list

	What to buy	Avoid	Alternatives
Carbs 60% of your diet	▶ Fresh fruit Dark green vegetables ▶ Whole grains (ie brown rice, millet, buckwheat) ▶ Brown bread ▶ Beans and pulses ▶ Crispbreads	▶ White bread/rice/ pasta/flour ▶ Sweetened breakfast cereals ▶ Potato chips ▶ Caffeine ▶ Cakes and biscuits ▶ Sugar	▶ Spelt, rice, buckwheat, millet, rye varieties ▶ Porridge or muesli ▶ High cocoa hot chocolate/herbal tea ▶ Dried fruit, honey or fruit juice
Fats 15–30% of your diet	▶ Oils – olive, rapeseed, canola, sesame seed ▶ Avocados ▶ Nuts (unsalted ▶ Seeds	▶ Margarine containing hydrogenated fat/ Lard or palm oil ▶ Fried food

▶ Fizzy drinks ▶ Alcohol | ▶ Olive, rapeseed, canola, sesame seed oils ▶ Steamed, grilled or poached ▶ Sparkling water with fruit juice or slices of fruit ▶ Sparkling water with fruit juice/ honey |
| **Protein** 10–15% of your diet | ▶ Oily fish (mackerel or salmon) ▶ Lean meat ▶ Eggs ▶ Butter ▶ Natural, live yoghurt | ▶ Fatty meat (ie streaky bacon, lamb) | ▶ Leaner meat (ie back bacon, chicken, turkey, beef) |

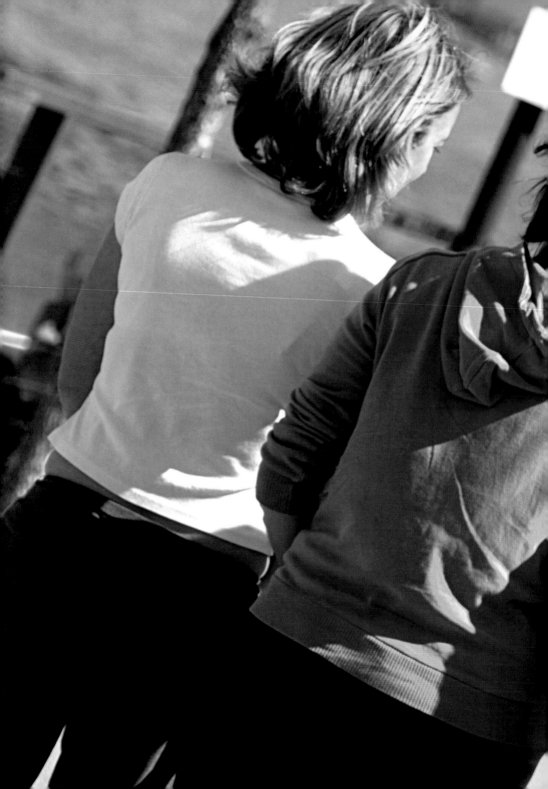

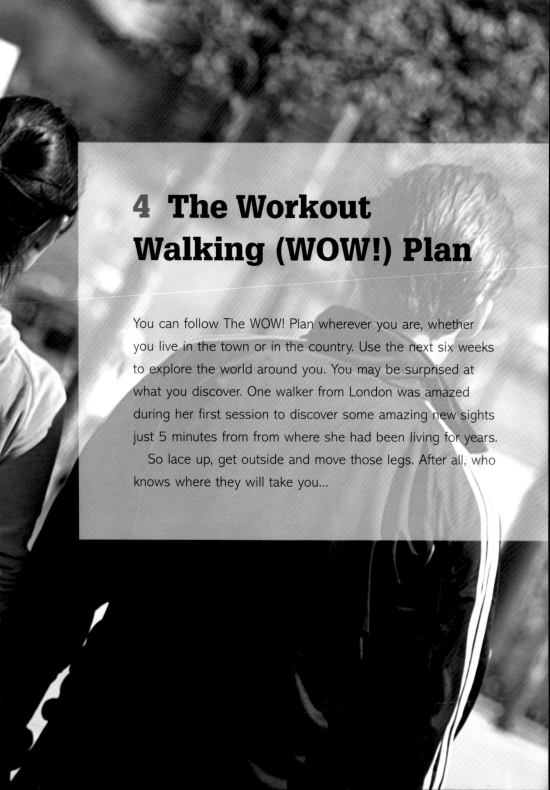

4 The Workout Walking (WOW!) Plan

You can follow The WOW! Plan wherever you are, whether you live in the town or in the country. Use the next six weeks to explore the world around you. You may be surprised at what you discover. One walker from London was amazed during her first session to discover some amazing new sights just 5 minutes from from where she had been living for years.

So lace up, get outside and move those legs. After all, who knows where they will take you...

Your 6-week Walking Plan

The weekly plans are easy to follow and each week new elements are introduced for you to bring in to your daily routine, while continuing with those you began in previous weeks. By the end of the 6 weeks you will have developed new skills and habits that will launch you towards the level of fitness that you have always wanted.

Try as far as possible to complete the daily walking sessions outlined in each weekly plan in one fell swoop. But where time really does not allow this, do 10–15 minute chunks whenever you can in order to complete the targets.

The weekly plans consist of:

► **Daily targets** These are to be completed on five days of the week (feel free to go out more often and for longer if you have the desire and the time). The focus is on daily rather than weekly targets for two reasons. Firstly, studies have shown that physical activity for moderate amounts of time on a regular basis is more beneficial than longer exercise sessions once or twice a week. Secondly, you need to concentrate on 'you' every single day – with a weekly target it is easier to brush it aside until the end of the week when you can then make up for all those days spent doing nothing! Reaching the goals you have set yourself requires a little effort every single day, not just every now and again.

The targets are measured by time which in turn is converted into steps, distance and calories burned at different speeds. The purpose of providing you with conversions at different speeds is to motivate you to push yourself harder as and when your health and fitness allow – you will see that as you walk faster, you will walk further and burn more calories. For example, if you start in Week 1 walking at 5 km (3 mph), the daily target of 20 minutes works out at 2,200 steps,

100 calories and 1.6 km (1 mile). Compare this to walking at 8 km/h (5 mph) (which you could well be doing by Week 6) when in 20 minutes you would be walking 3,740 steps, 2.7 km (1.7 miles) and burning 170 calories. So, whether it's miles walked or calories burned that interest you, this method will keep you motivated.

NB The number of calories that any one person burns depends on their weight and the distance travelled over a specific period of time. The heavier you are and the faster you walk, the more calories you will burn.

The conversion rates used in The WOW! Plan are based on an average weight in order to provide you with an easy way of measuring your progress.

▶ **Walking Plan** This starts at 20 minutes per day for at least 5 days per week, rising by 5 minutes each week to 45 minutes per day in Week 6. Treat these times as a minimum – if you fancy going out for longer periods, please do, you will get results even more quickly. Governments and health professionals recommend completing 10,000 steps a day, which takes about 1 hour depending on the speed you walk. We introduce a new walking technique each week, so that by the end of week six, you will have all you need for a thorough workout whenever you step out of the door.

▶ **Eating Plan** This is a fun way of eating more healthily. Each week you'll be set three new 'eating tasks' based on the dietary information covered in Chapters 1 and 3. Make these simple changes and by the end of Week 6 you will have laid the foundations for a healthy and nutritious diet.

How to structure your walking session

After Week 1, your session consists of three parts: Casting off, Toning up and Stretching. Toning up is the main part of your session and this is where you will incorporate the six amazing new walking techniques. You cannot do these techniques for long periods of time. Not only is it physically impossible, but it is simply not necessary. This is all about quality, not quantity. The best results come from practising the techniques for 2 minutes at a time. At first you may only be able to manage 10 or 15 seconds, but that's fine. You will soon get used to the exercises and be able to work up to the optimal time of 2 minutes.

Casting off

These first few minutes are absolutely essential to prepare your body for the movements that follow. They allow you the opportunity to leave behind any outside concerns that have been occupying your mind while giving your body a chance to warm up. During this period, do the first walking technique 4–4 Breathing (see page 80). It will become easier with practise and you will soon be able to incorporate both the breathing and WOW! techniques into your workout, rather than practising them separately. This type of deep, thoughtful breathing will help clear your mind and your lungs. Use this time to perfect your basic walking technique to iron out any problems that you may have (and didn't know about!) that are connected with the way you walk at the moment.

CASE STUDY **Jenny (36)**

Starting The WOW! Plan was one of the best things I've done. It made me think about what I really want from my life. Doing the techniques while walking was a bit strange at first but as I got used to them I did them automatically. It has given me the encouragement to go out on my own and walk for an hour. After all, I spend at least 5 hours a week watching soaps on TV and an hour a day walking is not a lot. The WOW! Plan is fun, enjoyable and a really positive thing for me.

Toning up

This is the workout phase of your walk, when you alternate between practising different WOW! techniques and walking normally. When choosing a technique, you will target a different area of your body for a bite-sized chunk of time. When performing a technique, do so for no more than 2 minutes at a time. Follow this with 2 minutes of walking normally, during which time you can relax and rest your muscles while clearing your lungs with 4–4 Breathing. Continue to switch between 2 minutes of a technique and 2 minutes of walking normally to get results.

Stretching

It is important, particularly when having exercised hard, to do a cool-down walk and some simple stretches (see page 104). The amount of time you stretch for depends on the length of time you have been exercising. Stretching in this way will help prevent injury, reduce soreness brought on by any build-up of lactic acid in your muscles, and make you more flexible.

Visualise what you should be doing, and you'll do it!

As you work through the WOW! techniques, you'll find that visualisation is a helpful way of learning what you should be doing and achieving it. When first trying to pick up something new, it's easy to become overwhelmed by all the things you have to remember and sometimes you can't see the wood for the trees. I suggest you read through the descriptions and look at the photos a few times before actually trying the technique yourself. As you're taking in this information, concentrate on visualising what you are trying to achieve, beginning by making yourself aware of the point on your body from which the movement starts and going on to imagine what you should be feeling.

You will find this approach particularly beneficial when you are learning to master the waist techniques.

Don't put pressure on yourself to do too much, or to master these techniques too quickly. There is no right or wrong amount of time in which to learn them. We are all different. Walking is, after all, about enjoying yourself and your surroundings so, even in the early stages, when you're concentrating on doing things right, don't forget to take some time out, let your mind wander and enjoy being in the open air!

Don't berate yourself, just get on with it!

If you miss a day's walking occasionally for whatever reason don't worry and absolutely DO NOT FEEL GUILTY. It is fine and to be expected. Just ensure that you make it up on other days so that you still reach your weekly targets.

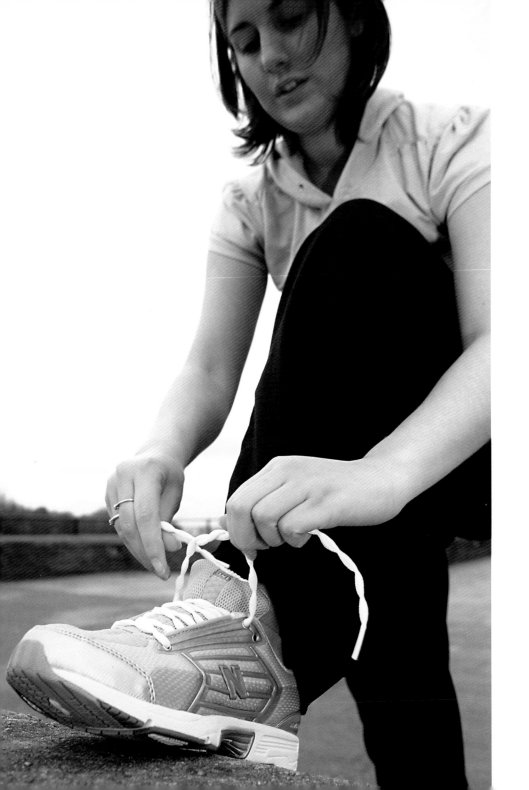

Basic walking technique and posture

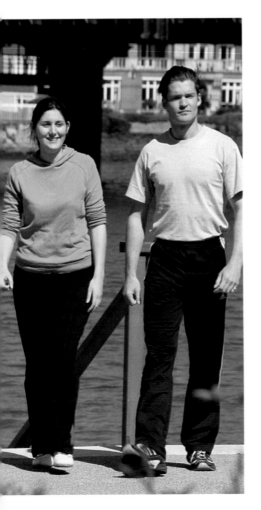

You've been walking practically all your life and you do it without thinking. But are you sure you are walking correctly? If any part of your body is misaligned, you could be harming your joints, suffering needless aches and pains and, worst of all, causing permanent damage to your body.

Walking properly is all about good posture. According to a study by the University of Miami, 90% of back problems could be prevented by adopting correct posture.

▶ Start by easing back those hunched shoulders and standing tall. Imagine you are being pulled up from the top of your head. If you normally stoop forward, you will find that your head falls back on your shoulders as soon as you start thinking about standing up straight.

▶ Try and hold in your abdominal muscles – imagine a piece of string pulling your belly button towards your spine. This helps protect your lower back as well as toning your abdominal muscles.

Heel to Toe Walking

▶ Keep your legs relaxed and loose.

▶ Do not stride out too far in front of your body, as this can put undue strain on your back.

▶ Do the Heel to Toe roll rather than walking flat-footed. When your heel strikes the ground (*see picture 1*), feel your foot rolling through the sole (*see picture 2*) until you can push off with your toes (*see picture 3*).

▶ Allow your arms to swing naturally in time with your stride.

▶ To prevent neck strain, keep your head up and look straight ahead.

▶ Be conscious of your breathing, taking deep breaths to provide your muscles with the oxygen they require to move.

You should find these steps simple, but sometimes retraining yourself out of bad habits can take a bit of effort. The main thing is to relax and stand tall and the rest will follow.

We're now ready to get started with Week 1.

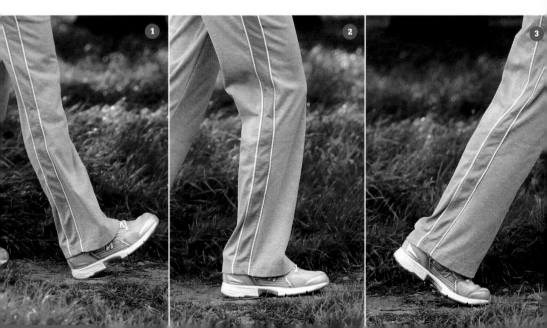

Week 1   Overview – what's happening?

Right, let's get cracking!

This week is about finding time for your new healthy lifestyle, developing a routine and discovering ways to improve what you already do. Your aim is to fit 20 minutes of walking into your daily routine, at least five times per week – you might struggle at first but with desire, dedication and determination, even the busiest person will find time to slot a walking session into their day. If you already do more than 20 minutes, that's great, continue to do more. From now on, though, start to monitor your walking time so that you can keep track of the calories you're burning off and the distance you're travelling – it's great fun and very rewarding to see how well you're doing!

Think about the way you walk during your outings this week. Look back at the correct basic walking technique and posture (page 76–77) to make sure that your movements are correct and that you're not putting undue strain on your body. The first thing you'll learn is simple 4–4 Breathing. Start practising 4–4 Breathing while you are out and about this week so it gradually becomes an integral part of your daily session.

You already know how important it is to drink enough water and keep salt to a minimum in your diet. Review Chapter 3 if you need reminding and watch out for your three weekly nutrition tasks.

Week 1 – Make the space

Daily Target = 20 mins	Speed	Steps	Distance	Calories
	5 km/h	2,200	1.6 km	100
	6.5 km/h	3,080	2.25 km	140
	8 km/h	3,740	2.7 km	170

Walking Plan

► This week find the time to fit 20 minutes into your day.
► Ensure your basic walking technique is correct – practise the Heel to Toe Roll (see page 77).
► Practise the 4–4 Breathing exercises.

Eating Plan

► Keep a food diary to find out where you can make improvements to your diet.
► Drink a glass of water every morning before eating or drinking anything else.
► Look for low-salt/salt-free versions of food.

Technique 1: 4–4 Breathing

We can live for weeks without food, days without water but only minutes without oxygen, the body's most vital ingredient. Yet we spend most of our lives taking in the bare minimum of oxygen for our body. Generally, we breathe so shallowly that we use as little as 20% of our lung capacity. That means that 80% of our lungs are either filled with stale air or not used at all.

Usually we are unaware of our breathing; after all, any changes needed in our breathing pattern are automatic and involuntary. With The WOW! Plan you will learn how to breathe more deeply, ensuring a fantastic and energising workout for your lungs.

4–4 Breathing helps fill your lungs and gives you maximum energy for your walking workout. Begin during the Casting off period of your session:

1   Start breathing in through your nose for four steps and breathing out through your mouth for the next four.
2   When breathing in, on the fourth stride fill your lungs as much as possible.
3   When breathing out, on the fourth stride really squeeze your lungs to empty them completely.
4   Keep your stomach muscles taut, so that just your lungs rise and fall with your breathing.

Breathing in such a way is powerful, so if you feel dizzy or unsteady, stop and breathe normally for a while. It may take a few days to feel totally comfortable with 4–4 Breathing, but if you persist, you will soon get used to it and feel much better for it. You may not have breathed in such a thoughtful manner before, and you will need to keep focused and check from time to time that you are taking four steps while inhaling and another four when exhaling. When filling your lungs, your posture improves, your shoulders go back, your head rises and you look 5cm (2 inches) taller ... and your brain is refreshed with the increased flow of oxygen!

When you start to use more energy by walking faster or uphill, increase the breathing rate to 3–3; that is breathing in for 3 strides and out for 3 strides, to ensure that your breathing rate matches the increased effort. Consciously changing your breathing pattern like this, before your body is actually forcing you to do so, should ensure that you always breathe easily without stress or breathlessness. Revert to 4–4 Breathing when your workload reduces. Continue with 3–3 Breathing for a few seconds after you slacken the pace or stop going uphill to allow your body time to adjust to the new workload.

4–4 Breathing is a great exercise for your stomach muscles, making them stronger so that they will keep you standing up straight, getting rid of those ageing, round shoulders.

4–4 Breathing checklist

- ▶ Breathe in through your nose (if you are unable to do so, because you have a cold or sinus problems, breathe in through your mouth) and out through your mouth.
- ▶ Check that you are breathing properly by placing your hand on your stomach and making sure it remains as still as possible, while your chest rises and falls with your breath. This is hard at first but worth mastering – it forces you to keep your stomach muscles taut, which will lead to a flatter stomach!
- ▶ If you feel dizzy, return to normal breathing.
- ▶ If 4–4 Breathing feels too fast and isn't stretching your lungs sufficiently, increase to 5–5 or 6–6, or whatever you are comfortable with. The objective of this breathing technique is to tone your lungs by using them fully, boost oxygen flow and improve posture
- ▶ Before you are about to walk uphill or increase your speed, change to 3–3 or even 2–2 Breathing to prevent breathlessness.

Week 2   Overview – what's happening?

By this week you should be used to the idea of fitting in some daily walking, have ironed out any problems with the way you normally walk and tried 4–4 Breathing.

It's time now to introduce you to the next technique: Heel Walking. This will help you tone up your legs and bottom. This week's daily target is 25 minutes of walking on at least 5 days. If you manage to do more than this, you will reap rewards more quickly.

How did you get on with keeping your food diary last week? It should have highlighted a few areas where you could improve, in addition to showing what you are already doing well. Now that you are more aware of what you are putting into your body, start thinking seriously about some of the poorer dietary choices you are making. Concentrate on how you can eliminate or reduce the unhealthy elements in your diet today in order boost your energy and performance and minimise health problems in later life.

Remember that the effects of The WOW! Plan are cumulative – each new good weekly habit is not a replacement for the previous week's habits, but an addition to them. So continue to start the day with a glass of water and to choose food with low salt content (Week 1) as well as bringing in this week's three new changes.

Have a great week!

Week 2 – Use it to lose it!

Daily Target = 25 mins	Speed	Steps	Distance	Calories
	5 km/h	2,750	2 km	125
	6.5 km/h	3,960	2.9 km	180
	8 km/h	4,620	3.4 km	210

Walking Plan		
	Casting off	**4 mins**
	Toning up	**18 mins**
	A Heel Walking x 2 mins	A x 5
	B Normal/4–4 Breathing x 2 mins	B x 4
	Stretching (see pages 104–107)	**3 mins**

Eating Plan	
	▶ Replace at least three simple carbohydrates with complex alternatives, eg brown rice, pasta and bread instead of the white versions (see Shopping List on page 67 for ideas).
	▶ Reduce the amount of tea/coffee you drink to two cups per day (eliminate if possible), replacing with glasses of water.
	▶ Reduce your intake of sugar – use honey, dried or fresh fruit to add sweetness to food.

Technique 2: Heel Walking

The forward motion comes from your front leg, which is pulling your body forward. This technique works the back of your legs and buttocks.

When you are Heel Walking correctly, it will feel almost as if someone is pushing your bottom, propelling you forward quite fast. The resulting steps that you take are fairly short and choppy and you will become more upright. As with all the WOW! techniques, Heel Walking encourages very good posture.

When performing this technique correctly, you will feel a tension all the way up the back of your leg, from your calves to your hamstring and bottom. You will really feel your legs working hard and toning up at every step. One sign that you have mastered this powerful first technique is that when you revert to walking normally you will feel like you are doing absolutely nothing!

So this week, see how you get on with Heel Walking, while continuing with the basic Heel to Toe Roll as well as the 4–4 Breathing. Remember that the new things you learn each week must be incorporated into what you have picked up in previous weeks, so that by the end of the 6-week period you have a whole set of positive, healthy habits that you automatically do every day.

When you have completed your walking target this week you will have:

▶ Walked the length of 92.5 football (soccer) pitches at 5 km (3 mph)!
▶ Burned off 6 bottles of beer at 6.5 km (4 mph)!
▶ Melted away the equivalent of more than 4.5 Mars Bars at 8.5 km (5 mph)!

Congratulations. You have made great progress over the last couple of weeks. Getting started is often the hardest part and that is exactly what you have done. You should already be feeling happier and more energetic. Remember that for every day you follow this plan, you are increasing your life expectancy. If you miss a day, don't worry. Just add any missed time to later sessions in the week.

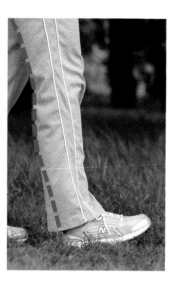

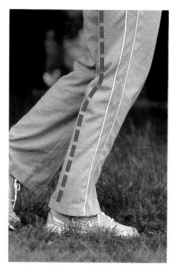

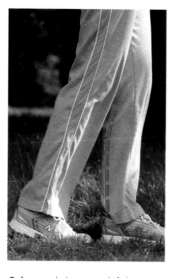

1 Start with your right leg. Stand up straight and when your right heel strikes the ground at the start of the step, tense the back of your right (front) leg slightly and use this tension to pull yourself forward from your heel.

2 Allow your left (back) leg to simply follow. It is important that you do not straighten your right leg (the front leg that is pulling you forward) even though you are tensing it.

3 As you bring your left leg forward, it will become the front leg. As your left foot strikes the ground, tense your left leg muscles to pull your body forward, bringing with it a relaxed right (back) leg. Your right leg returns to the front; repeat from step 1.

NB Remember to shorten your stride at the outset and to keep the toes of your back foot relaxed so you do not push off with them – your legs must now do all the work. Most importantly, relax and keep breathing!

Week 3 Overview – what's happening?

We're really starting to make headway now.

This week, your daily walking target has risen to 30 minutes. If you're managing to fit in more than your targets, are you keeping a note of the total amount that you're doing? At the end of the 6 weeks, use the results chart on page 115 to see how far you've walked and exactly how many calories you've burned off. You might find that you've walked from London to Paris!

I wonder how you got on with Heel Walking last week. It should be feeling quite natural to you now – keep practising the technique on a daily basis for 2 minutes at a time. Each time you start Heel Walking, you should feel yourself immediately standing more upright and improving your posture. Enjoy the feeling of your legs becoming stronger and leaner with every stride you take.

This week, you will keep working on your legs but will also be shown how to start busting all that stored energy around your waist! First learn how our waist techniques differ from the leg exercises and then get going with the third great walking technique, Waist Pushing. Don't worry if it feels strange to begin with – it should. It will become easier and smoother in no time at all.

On the dietary front, you should now be starting to choose more nutritious carbohydrates, opting for slower-burning, complex types rather than the simpler, less nutritious ones. Why not start making a note of the credits and debits going in and out of your Health Account (see page 56)? Don't forget to keep up the nutrition tasks from Weeks 1 and 2 while completing this week's three new ones.

Week 3 – Melt away your middle

Daily Target = 30 mins	Speed	Steps	Distance	Calories
	5 km/h	3,300	2.4 km	150
	6.5 km/h	4,620	3.4 km	210
	8km/h	5,500	4 km	250

Walking Plan		
	Casting off	**3 mins**
	Toning up	**24 mins**
	A Waist Pushing x 2 mins	A x 3
	Normal/4–4 Breathing x 2 mins	
	B Heel Walking x 2 mins	B x 3
	Stretching (see pages 104–107)	**3 mins**

Eating Plan

- ▶ Read food labels, leaving behind items with high saturated fat, sugar or salt content.
- ▶ Eat 3 portions of Omega 3 Fatty Acids (see list on page 62).
- ▶ When cooking, avoid frying food in oil; instead experiment with other methods such as baking, steaming, grilling or poaching.

Feel the movement

To tackle the troublesome area around your middle when walking you need to twist your waist to move your body forward. Your legs should remain relaxed, simply following where they are led by the rotation of the waist.

Like anything new, these movements will seem odd at first. But be patient, because with a little effort and persistence they become familiar very quickly. Believe me, it's worth persevering – they work absolute wonders. These unusual movements get your body moving in ways it's not used to; they massage your internal organs while busting excess weight around your abdomen, leading to a more toned midriff and a stronger back. They help strengthen your body core, which has led people to compare the WOW! walking techniques to Pilates.

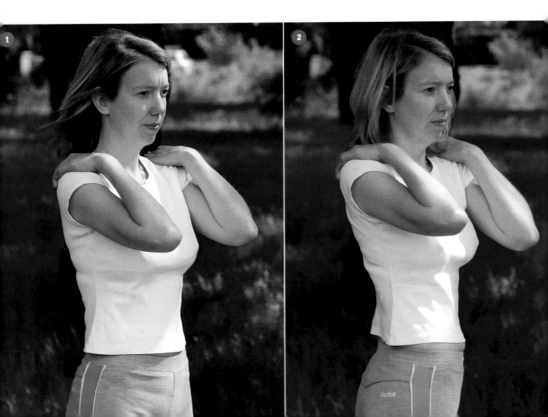

When doing these waist techniques, be sure to keep your legs and ankles relaxed: your legs move forward as a result of the waist movement and not through any effort of their own. Your arms should move naturally, merely providing a counterbalance to your leg movements. If you swing your arms more vigorously, the exaggerated movement will help propel you forward, making it easier on your middle and reducing the energy expended by your waist.

First let's see what these movements will feel like:

▶ Stand up straight and keep your body still. Keep your shoulders steady by holding them with your hands – left hand on left shoulder, right hand on right shoulder (*see picture 1*).
▶ Slowly twist at your waist, making sure that only your waist moves.

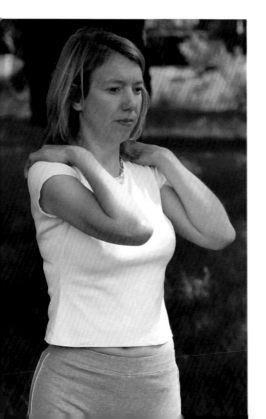

Most of us are stiff in this area, so it may take a little time before your waist moves separately from the rest of your torso. It is important that you do this gently at first to give the whole area a chance to loosen up (*see pictures 2 & 3*). Doesn't it feel good to get that whole area moving?

Many of us suffer from lower-back weakness and pain and the waist techniques, if done properly, can loosen and strengthen this area. Make sure you are protecting your back by holding your stomach in and imagining a piece of string pulling your belly button towards your spine. This should prevent any back discomfort by realigning your spine in the correct position.

Technique 3: Waist Pushing

With this third technique, the forward motion comes from the rotation of your waist. This technique will tighten your abdomen and loosen your lower back. Firstly, make sure that your legs are perfectly relaxed, because it will be the power from your waist (not your legs) that moves your body forward.

Start by moving forward with your right leg. Waist Pushing is actually very simple, but because it feels rather awkward at first, it can appear complicated. When first learning the technique, people have described it as a feeling akin to walking like a model down a catwalk. Your feet fall along the same line in front of your body: in fact, at the outset, your feet may even cross each other, with your toes pointing inwards, as if you are

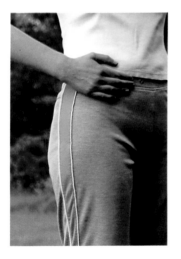
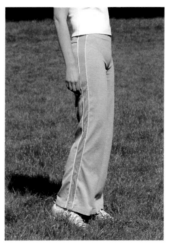
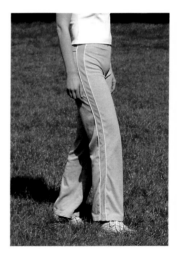

1 Focus on a point on the right side of your waist.

2 From this point rotate your waist anti-clockwise (left) and allow this movement (push) to bring your right leg forward.

3 Remember to keep your right leg relaxed, not pushing off with your toes.

pigeon-toed. The pigeon-toed phase often lasts as little as a couple of minutes. Once you start to feel what the movement is all about, your feet stop crossing each other and start naturally falling along the same line in front of your body. When this happens you will love the sensation of really shifting all that stagnant energy around your waist as it propels you forward.

When you have completed your walking target this week you will have:

- ▶ Crossed the famous 'coat hanger' Sydney Harbour Bridge (believe me, it's a long way, I've done it!) almost 10 times at 5 km/h (3 mph)!
- ▶ Walked the equivalent of the height of London's BT Tower 84 times at 6.5 km/h (4 mph)!!
- ▶ Melted away the effects of 2 Mars Bars, a bowl of pasta and 2 slices of pizza at 8 km/h (5 mph)!!!

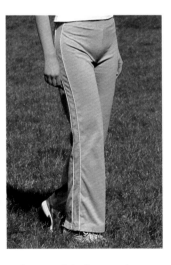

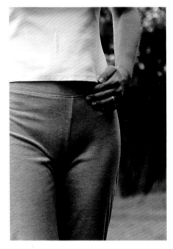

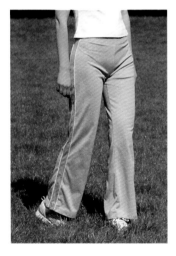

4 As your right foot touches the ground, repeat on the other side.

5 Focus on a point on the left side of your waist. From this point rotate your waist clockwise (right).

6 Allow the movement of your waist to push your left foot forward to complete the second step. Repeat stages 1–6.

Week 4 — Overview – what's happening?

You are really starting to build up healthy habits now. Are there any particular lifestyle changes that you find easier to adopt than others? Perhaps you're picking up the walking movements easily but finding it difficult to change your eating habits? Whatever your concerns, don't worry. You are changing the patterns of a lifetime so expect a few bumps along the way. The main thing is to keep going because these very small, individual changes will make a big difference in your life.

This week's walking target is 35 minutes. Have you found that you are treating these times as a minimum and in actual fact going out for longer and longer periods? If this is the case, remember to keep a tally of the amount you walk so that you can keep track of your cumulative calories, steps, miles or time.

So far you've learned about 4–4 Breathing, Heel Walking and Waist Pushing and should by now be feeling fairly comfortable with all three. While you continue with these, you're now going to focus again on those legs and behind with the fourth technique, Heel Pulling. You're developing quite a fitness repertoire! Don't confine these techniques to your daily sessions – start using them in your everyday walking around the office or house to get results even faster.

If you haven't begun to do so, now's the time to start taking a healthy breakfast every morning ... good luck with the three eating tasks this week.

Make sure you're still doing the tasks from previous weeks. You'll have seen how much better you feel for them – so keep them up! Remember the goals you're working towards. If you feel like wavering at any point, remind yourself that persistence is the key. Don't let anything stand in the way of you and success.

Week 4 – Tone those legs

Daily Target = 35 mins	Speed	Steps	Distance	Calories
	5 km/h	3,850	2.8 km	175
	6.5 km/h	5,500	4 km	250
	8 km/h	6,380	4.6 km	290

Walking plan	**Casting off**	**4 mins**
	Toning up	**28 mins**
	A Heel Pulling x 2 mins	A x 3
	Normal/4–4 Breathing x 2 mins	
	B Waist Pushing x 2 mins	B x 3
	Normal/4–4 Breathing x 2 mins	
	C Heel Walking x 2	C x 1
	Normal/4–4 Breathing x 2 mins	
	Stretching (see pages 104–107)	**3 mins**

Eating Plan	▶ Add colour to your diet by eating something green, something red and something citrus every day to guarantee a good mix of vitamins and minerals.
	▶ Take breakfast every day this week, trying some of the healthy options suggested on page 67.
	▶ Think carefully before eating any junk food and replace with healthier options.

Technique 4: Heel Pulling

Heel Pulling is an extended version of Heel Walking, where your legs do all the work and your waist is allowed to relax. If you suffer or have suffered in the past from a groin injury, take Heel Pulling gently at first to make sure that you don't overdo it. This technique works your thigh and groin, and tones the back of your legs and bottom.

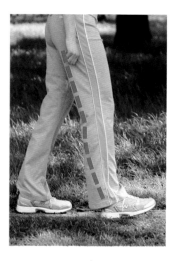
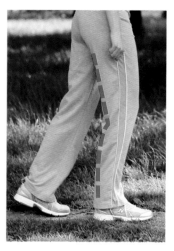
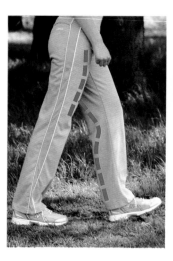

1 Begin by Heel Walking. Strike your right heel on the ground close to your body, tensing the back of your leg and pulling positively against the ground to move your body forward.

2 As your right leg passes under your body, your left leg comes forward and repeats the same movement. You should feel the backs of your legs and your bottom working hard at every stride.

3 Now introduce the Heel Pulling element. This time, when your right foot passes under your body and becomes the trailing foot, keep it on the ground slightly longer than normal. You will feel a tension in the front of your right (trailing) thigh and groin, as this area is stretched. Repeat on the other side.

Essentially, you are holding yourself back by keeping your back foot on the ground, which means your leading leg has to work harder to pull your body forward and keep walking at the same speed. When Heel Pulling, your back foot leaves the ground slightly flatter than normal, from the ball of the foot rather than the toes. This all-round leg technique is a very effective use of your muscles, exercising the back of your leg and bottom at the start of the step, and toning your thigh and stretching your groin at the end of the stride. It is one of the most effective techniques. When you have completed your walking target this week you will have:

▶ Burned off 17 cans of fizzy drink or more than 9 cheeseburgers AND walked more than 1 marathon or covered more than 103 laps around an Olympic outdoor athletics track, at 5 km/h (3 mph)!

▶ Completed 1½ marathons or walked the equivalent of the height of the Hoover Dam in Colorado, USA 265 times AND burned off 23 gin and tonics or nearly 18 slices of pizza, at 6.5 km (4 mph)!!

▶ Walked the height of the Eiffel Tower more than 214 times or ⅙ of the length of the Grand Canyon AND melted away 0.5 kg (1 lb 4 oz) of body fat (more if you are eating fewer calories than before) or 9 Big Macs and 1 glass of white wine, at 8 km (5 mph)!!!

This is just the beginning. If you walk just 3.2 km (2 miles) 5 days per week throughout the year, you will have done the equivalent of walking from London to Paris AND back PLUS travelling from New York to Philadelphia PLUS completing 18 miles of a marathon! It soon adds up.

If losing weight is one of your goals, you need to use more calories than you consume. If you indulge one day, that's okay, but make sure you make amends by exercising more. As you become fitter, start picking up the intensity when you're walking to make your heart work harder and your body burn more fat.

Week 5 | Overview – what's happening?

How did you get on with Heel Pulling? Hopefully you'll appreciate the way you can feel the whole of your leg working and toning up at every step. If you've also managed to eat a healthy breakfast every day, you'll have felt a resulting positive increase in your energy levels. Once you feel immediate benefits from a change in behaviour, it becomes easier to make it a permanent feature in your life.

This week you're aiming for 40 minutes of walking per day, broken into two parts if necessary, but preferably done all together. It's an ideal amount of time, for example, to fit into your lunch break.

This week is also the time to step it up with a more advanced walking technique – Waist Pulling. You will find it is a great complement to the waist technique you have already learned, Waist Pushing, because it targets different muscles. When you use both techniques together in a session, your waist, abdomen and back will get a really thorough workout.

Keep up all those healthy eating habits and experiment with some foods you haven't included before. Have fun discovering new, (hopefully tasty), things. If you drink alcohol, your new healthy living regime has may well have encouraged you to cut back.

Week 5 – Use it to improve it

Daily Target = 40 mins	Speed	Steps	Distance	Calories
	5 km/h	4,400	3.2 km	200
	6.5 km/h	6,160	4.5 km	280
	8 km/h	7,260	5.3 km	330

Walking Plan		
	Casting off	**4 mins**
	Toning up	**32 mins**
	A Waist Pulling x 2 mins	A x 2
	Normal/4–4 Breathing x 2 mins	
	B Heel Pulling x 2 mins	B x 2
	Normal/4–4 Breathing x 2 mins	
	C Waist Pushing x 2 mins	C x 2
	Normal/4–4 Breathing x 2 mins	
	D Heel Walking x 2 mins	D x 2
	Normal/4–4 Breathing x 2 mins	
	Stretching (see pages104–107)	**4 mins**

Eating Plan

▶ Fill up on healthy foods such as fruit and vegetables. This will reduce your desire for sugary or fatty foods.

▶ Try 3 foods you have never had before.

▶ Reduce your alcohol intake – why not cut it out your week completely?

Technique 5: Waist Pulling

You will feel the effects of this exercise higher up than with the first waist technique, in your external oblique muscles as well as your back. This is a more advanced version of Waist Pushing, because the waist rotation is greater. With Waist Pulling, you rotate the waist in the same direction as for Waist Pushing, but this time you start the waist rotation from the opposite side to the leg that you are moving forward.

Now is a good time to remind yourself of the importance of using visualisation to learn new techniques. Visualisation is particularly important for the waist techniques. Once you have read the instructions below, take a moment to visualise what you are aiming to achieve and the points from which to start the movement before going any further.

One way of describing the feeling you get when doing this technique is

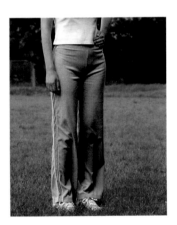 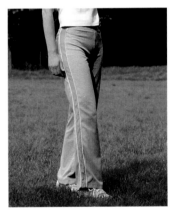 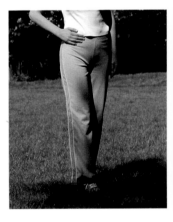

1 Focus on a point on the left side of your waist.

2 From this point rotate your waist anti-clockwise (left/backwards), moving your right leg forward simultaneously. As your right foot lands, repeat on the other side.

3 Focus on a point on the right side of your waist, and from this point rotate your waist clockwise (right/backwards).

of your hip being pushed backwards. For example, in order to bring your right leg forward, you concentrate on a point on the left side of your waist and it's at this point that you feel your left hip pushing backwards. You may find this easier to grasp than thinking about your waist rotating anti-clockwise and pulling your right leg forward.

When you begin this technique it will feel even more exaggerated than when you started Waist Pushing. Rest assured – it really won't be long before you get to grips with it, and it has got to grips with you!

NB The waist rotation is greater with this technique so your body will rotate slightly on the ball of your foot during the movement. This causes a slight twisting at the knee. This is a more advanced technique than the previous three so if you have any knee problems you should take it very gently at first in order to give your knees time to adjust. If you feel any pain or discomfort, stop immediately and return to normal walking.

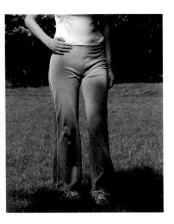

When you have completed your walking target this week you will have:

▶ Burned off nearly 6 doughnuts at 5 km/h (3 mph)!
▶ Melted away the calories of nearly 13 glasses of dry white wine at 6.5 km/h (4 mph)!!
▶ Walked the height of the London Eye more than 183 times at 8 km/h (5 mph)!!!

4 This movement will pull your left foot forward, thereby completing the second step. Repeat stages 1–4.

Week 6   Overview – what's happening?

Congratulations! You've made it to Week 6.

You have achieved a great deal in a very short amount of time and opened up endless possibilities. With good habits, a positive attitude and improving health, you can forge ahead and fulfill your potential. As you reach your goals, why not make some more? What you're achieving now is just the beginning – you can reach whatever you aim for. So capitalise on the momentum you've built up and strive to attain ever higher goals.

The WOW! Plan finishes with a daily walking target of 45 minutes. As your energy levels have been boosted throughout the weeks and you have learned new ways to make your walking fun and challenging, you're probably more than happy to go out for this amount of time and possibly longer.

Now that you have learned the basic posture and walking technique, 4–4 Breathing, Heel Walking, Waist Pushing, Heel Pulling and Waist Pulling, you're ready for the big one. The Waist Buster is a real phenomenon! You won't need to do it for very long (believe me, you won't be able to) to achieve great results.

Your body is probably rewarding you in many ways as you have been boosting your Health Account over these past few weeks. With the last three eating tasks, combined with everything else you have done in The WOW! Plan, you'll be even closer to the life you deserve.

Week 6 – Make it count

Daily Target = 45 mins	Speed	Steps	Distance	Calories
	5 km	4,950	3.6 km	225
	6.5 km	7,040	5.1 km	320
	8 km	8,360	6.1 km	380

Walking Plan		
	Casting off	**5 mins**
	Toning up	**36 mins**
	Waist Buster x 20 secs at least 5 times	
	A Heel Walking x 2 mins	A x 2
	Normal/4–4 Breathing x 2 mins	
	B Waist Pushing x 2 mins	B x 2
	Normal/4–4 Breathing x 2 mins	
	C Heel Pulling x 2 mins	C x 3
	Normal/4–4 Breathing x 2 mins	
	D Waist Pulling x 2 mins	D x 2
	Normal/4–4 Breathing x 2 mins	
	Stretching (see pages 104–107)	**4 mins**

Eating Plan	
	▶ Include at least 3 superfoods in your meals such as blueberries, ginger, garlic and sprouts.
	▶ Cut out all unhealthy snacks.
	▶ Have a look at the Shopping List (see page 67) and make any final healthy substitutes.

Technique 6: The Waist Buster

This will set your abdomen, stomach and external oblique muscles on fire! The Waist Buster requires you to keep your mid-section still while you do the first waist technique, Waist Pushing. This is an incredibly powerful exercise. Don't try the Waist Buster until you have thoroughly warmed up, either in the middle or towards the end of your workout. And don't expect to do this for long – if you manage 10 seconds you're doing well! Keep your stomach muscles taut throughout this technique.

Do the Waist Buster for as long as you can bear (no matter how short this is) and keep going back to it between normal walking. You will soon start to see results right across your middle section. This week, slot 20-second bouts of the Waist Buster into your daily sessions between the other WOW! techniques.

When you have completed your walking target this week you will have:

▶ Burned off 12½ slices of thick bread, at 5 km/h (3 mph)!
▶ Burned off 3 Big Macs and a glass of dry white wine, at 6.5 km/h (4 mph)!!
▶ Burned off 8¼ Mars Bars, at 8 km/h (5 mph) !!!

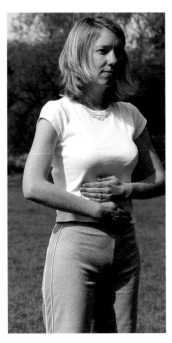

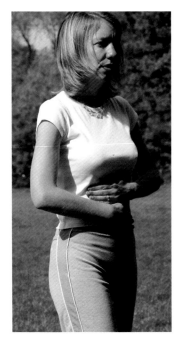

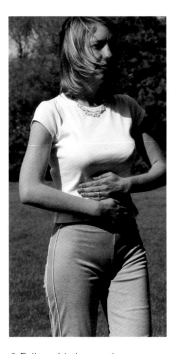

1 Start by Heel Walking. Keep your abdomen and stomach muscles taut. Do this by imagining that there are three vertical rods passing through your stomach muscles, one on the left side, another on the right, and the third passing through your navel. The purpose of these imaginary rods is to keep your torso as still as possible.

2 Now you're ready for the hard bit. Keeping your stomach still and taut, start Technique 3, Waist Pushing. Rotate your waist anti-clockwise (left) from a point on the right side, to bring your right foot forward.

3 Follow this by rotating your waist clockwise (right) from a point on its left side to bring your left foot forward. Remember that the purpose of this exercise is to keep you mid-section still while you attempt to rotate your waist. You will find that your waist muscles will try to resist and your whole midriff will feel as if it is on fire!

The stretches

If you have done anything more than a gentle walk, you should cool down and stretch your muscles before finishing your workout. When your muscles work hard, lactic acid can build up in your legs, leading to soreness and muscle tightness. Stretching alleviates this problem by breaking down the lactic acid and releasing it into the bloodstream, leaving you with relaxed, loose muscles. (You might consider doing a few stretches when you have finished your Casting off period if you are about to embark on a particularly long and arduous Toning up session. If you choose to do this, make sure that you only stretch once your body and muscles have warmed up because stretching when they are cold can lead to injury).

Stretching is important for the following reasons:

- ▶ It makes you more flexible.
- ▶ It helps your body get rid of toxins, leaving you with more energy.
- ▶ It eases the discomfort of tight, sore muscles.
- ▶ It reduces the risk of injury.
- ▶ Loosening your muscles improves your posture – you may appear thinner and taller.
- ▶ It can ease stress and make you feel better in yourself.
- ▶ It feels really good!

You are probably already familiar with some stretches. There are many to choose from; the stretches on the following pages are the most appropriate for ending a walking session. They target the muscles that you will have worked in your sessions and can all be done standing up (so you won't need to sit down by the side of the road!).

When performing these stretches, make sure you do not bounce because this can cause injury.

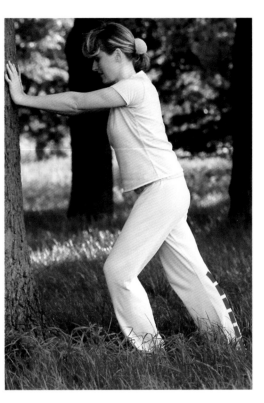 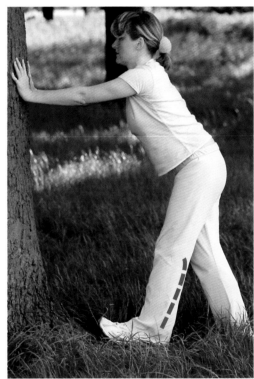

1 The calves Stand about 30cm (12inches) away from a wall, bench or tree and place your hands against the support and lean forward. Step back with the right leg, keeping it straight and press the right heel down. Feel the tension in the right calf. Hold for 15 seconds and repeat on the other side.

2 The calves (stretches the muscle under the calf). Stand about 30cm (12inches) away from a wall, bench or tree. Place your hands against the wall and lean forward. Step back with the right leg, keeping it straight. With your right leg stretched back, transfer your weight by pushing down on your left leg, relaxing and bending your right leg. Point the toes of your left foot up. Hold for 15 seconds and repeat on the other side. Feel the tension in your left calf.

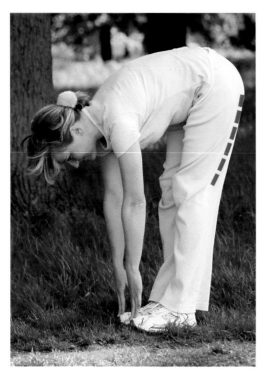

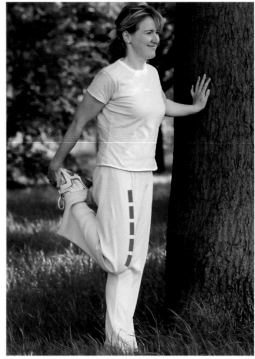

3 The backs of your thighs (hamstrings)

Stand with your feet shoulder-width apart, knees soft (slightly bent), toes pointing straight ahead. Bend forward at the hips and reach your hands towards your ankles. Feel for mild tension in the backs of your legs. Hold for 15 seconds and repeat on the other side.

4 The fronts of your thighs (quadriceps)

Stand holding a wall, bench or tree for balance. Bend your right knee up behind you as you reach back and grasp your right ankle with your right hand, keeping your knee close to your body. Pull your right heel towards your buttocks, keeping your back straight. Feel for mild tension in the front of your thigh. Hold for 15 seconds and repeat on the other side.

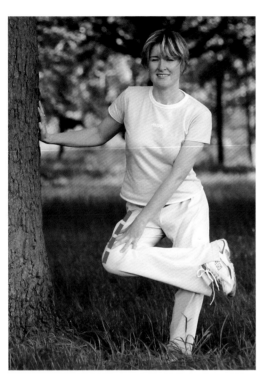

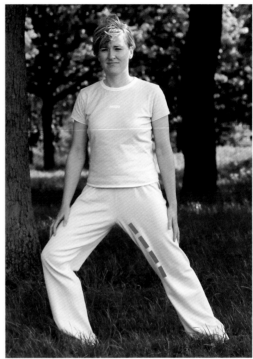

5 Outside thigh Hold on to a bench or wall, sideways on. Cross your right leg over your left leg and 'sit'. You will feel a stretch on the outside of the crossed over leg. Hold for 15 seconds and repeat on the other side. As you get fitter and more supple, you will be able to sit deeper.

6 Inner thigh Spread your legs about two shoulder widths apart. Bend your right leg, keeping your left leg straight. Keep the toe of your left (straight) leg pointing forwards in front of your body, while the toe of your right (bent) leg should point outwards to your right side. You will feel a stretch on the inner thigh of your straight leg. Hold for 15 seconds and repeat on other side. As you become fitter and more flexible, you will be able to 'dip' more deeply.

CASE STUDY **Camilla (35)**

....

I am generally walking for more than the suggested amount of time –
20–25 minutes morning and evening and. I definitely feel more energised
and am drinking plenty of water and eating lots of fresh things. I feel lighter
and more toned. I am smoking less too and feel better for it. I have done the
stretches suggested and can now touch my toes. I have always been a
flexible person, if overweight and exhausted.

I have lost 3.4kg (7½ lbs) and have lost inches off my waist. I have
started yoga again after a few years and am surprised to see how supple
I am. I feel strong and have found walking to be the ultimate stress-buster.
I was walking with a male colleague of mine who is a former athlete and he
said that I walk faster than any woman he knows – I now find it quite
difficult to walk at a normal speed. This has ultimately reflected upon my
diet as I now eat fruit for breakfast, have cut out unsafe fats, eat soya
protein during the week and think of meat as a weekend treat.

I don't expect these things to make all my problems disappear but
I feel that everything has a direct impact on my mood and outlook and
can alleviate feelings of fatigue and depression. I feel more in control of
my metabolism, and general well-being than I ever have and it's easy!
I wish others could realise that it is all within very easy reach.

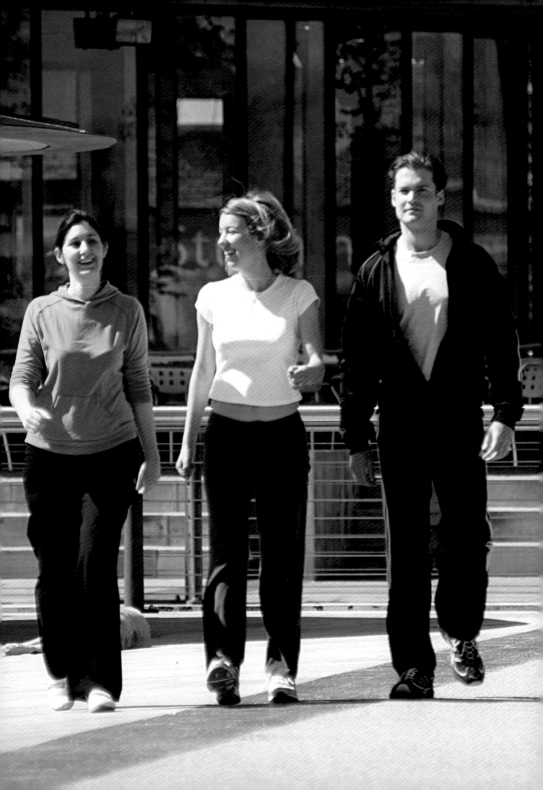

What next?

You've completed 6 weeks of walking and healthy eating. You should now be both willing and able to do all sorts of things that you may not have been able to do 6 weeks ago. The world is your oyster!

Take a look at your food diary from Week 1 and see how things have changed. If there are changes still to make (it doesn't matter if there are, in fact it would be surprising if there weren't), follow the example set by The WOW! Plan and make one or two changes each week until you've cracked it.

Make the most of your investment in the WOW! techniques by using them every day during dedicated walks as well as on short trips to the corner shop or the dry cleaners. The more you practise them, the easier they will become and it will increasingly be unnecessary to even think about the techniques because you'll be doing them naturally. You have a great opportunity to make every bit of walking you do each day into the very best it can be for you, working your heart and muscles in a safe yet effective way and melting away any excess body fat you may have.

You will never grow out of these techniques – they just keep on working, however fit you become. As your fitness levels increase, push yourself further by walking faster (remember Abba's 'Waterloo', or Meatloaf's 'Dead Ringer for Love' if you're really going for it) and including hilly terrain. If you live in a city on level ground, perhaps you can travel out to steeper ground at weekends to push your body further (only when it's ready, of course).

Before you opened this book you knew nothing about the six amazing ways that make every walk into a workout:

- ▶ 4–4 Breathing (page 77)
- ▶ Heel Walking (page 84)
- ▶ Waist Pushing (page 90)
- ▶ Heel Pulling (page 94)

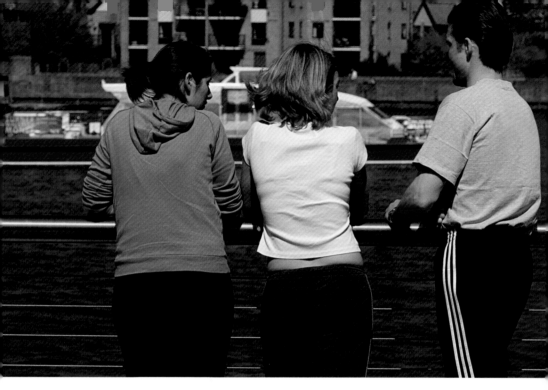

► Waist Pulling (page 98)
► The Waist Buster (page 102)

Over the last 6 weeks, walking 5 days per week, you have achieved the following:

► At 5 km (3 mph)	4,875 calories	78.5 km (48.75 miles)
► At 6.5 km (6.5 mph)	7,300 calories	117.5 (73 miles)
► At 8 km (5 mph)	8,150 calories	131 km (81.5 miles)

Of course, this doesn't take into account any extra you have been doing; only you know the correct total for you. And remember that if you are overweight, you will have burned more calories than those in our chart. Check over the page to see what your totals (so far) equate to. Keep these totals going so that by the end of the year you can see what you have managed to achieve over a whole year.

In the next chapter you'll discover all sorts of ways to make your walking even more fun, exciting and challenging!

Distance and calorie charts

There's no better motivation than seeing at a glance exactly how hard you have been working.

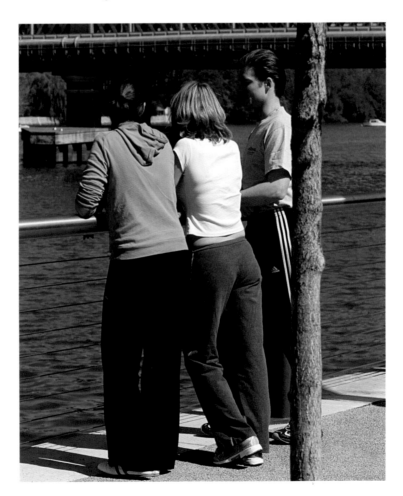

How far have you walked?

What	Measurement (in metres)
Soccer pitch (length)	100
Hoover Dam, USA (height)	221
Eiffel Tower (height)	322
Running track (one lap)	400
Empire State Building (height)	443
Sydney Harbour Bridge (overall length)	1,149
Golden Gate Bridge (overall length)	2,824
London to Paris	342,781
Grand Canyon, USA	450,604
Sydney to Melbourne	706,483
Lands End to John O'Groats	1,400,091

What have you burned off?

Food and drink	Calories
Slice thick bread	90
Glass dry white wine	110
Cappuccino	150
Can of fizzy drink (soda)	160
Doughnut	175
Slice of pizza	220
Chocolate bar	230
Cheeseburger	300
Bowl pasta (no sauce)	320

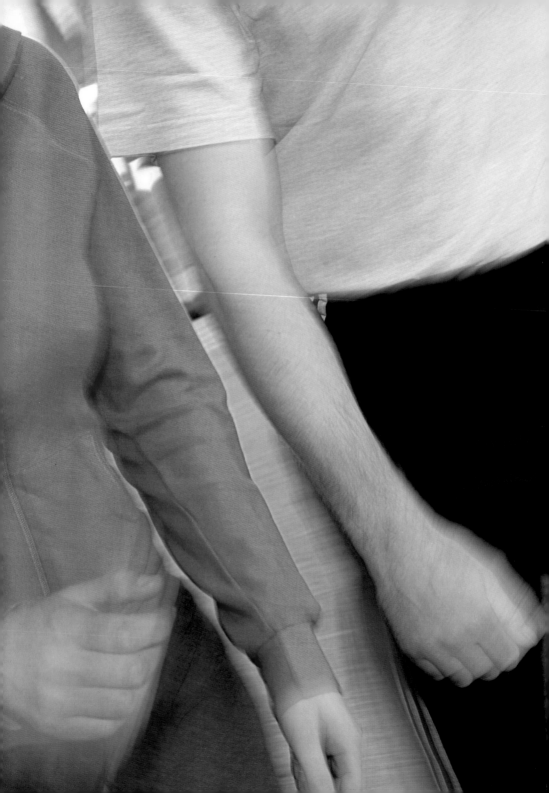

5 Having fun

This chapter should give you lots of ideas on how to add spice to your walking workouts and so keep your motivation as high as possible. It also introduces you to group walking, and gives tips on how to set up a walking group yourself. You might even like to think about pushing yourself further for longer and train for a distance walking event.

Making time fly

Even the most dedicated walker can feel stale sometimes. Here are a few ideas to help you keep you keen:

- ▶ If you're lucky enough to have a Heart Rate Monitor, try to spend longer in your target heart zone or time yourself over a set distance to see if you can complete it in a faster time than before.
- ▶ When wearing a pedometer, increase the number of steps you take at regular intervals to keep pushing yourself forward.
- ▶ Keep a record of your cumulative distance, steps, calories and/or time spent exercising and use the chart above to see where you have walked to and what you've walked off.
- ▶ Vary the route that you walk from country paths, to riverside walks to parks and city streets. Wherever you live, there are options available to you, even if it means travelling to discover a new area.
- ▶ Walk between two points that you would normally cover by car or public transport and be surprised by what you find. This can be particularly fun if you live in a city that has an underground transport system, if you walk between stations above ground. You may be surprised at how close many of the stations actually are.
- ▶ Go on a treasure hunt. Run through the alphabet, having to find or see something each day that begins with a new letter ie apple (outside a grocer's), bus, cat etc.
- ▶ Count things along the way, such as red cars, birds or even Christmas trees at the right time of year!
- ▶ If you are walking with another person or people, why not play the old favourite, I-Spy? If you're walking fast, you had better choose something far enough in front so you haven't passed it before anyone has had a chance to guess it!

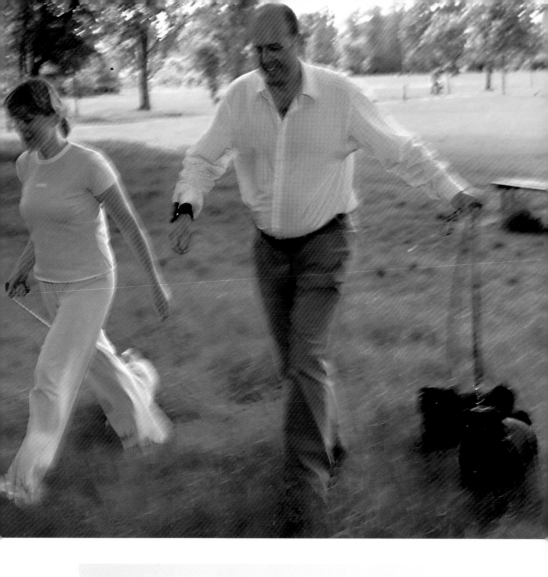

Dog walking

Taking your dog out on one of your walking sessions is a terrific way
to meet people as strangers feel comfortable talking about your dog.
Animals have the power to break down barriers in this way, putting
people at ease. You might even meet someone who is interested in
setting up a walking group with you (see page 122).

Walking on your own

With most sports and activities, you are dependent on other people to take part. With walking, you need not be reliant on others; instead you can enjoy total freedom to go out when, where and with or without others, depending on your situation and how you feel. Whether you fit your daily walking into your schedule is entirely down to you and no-one else. Walking allows you to take responsibility for your health and positively influence your life.

Going for a walk on your own is a wonderful opportunity to reflect on matters affecting your life and gain fresh perspective on issues you may be currently facing. Not only are you giving yourself space and time to work things out away from the stress and noise of daily life, but you are doing so while improving your fitness and boosting your energy – and this will help you think more clearly.

Equally, going for a walk on your own allows you to shut down your mind completely and savour the moment and surroundings as you speed through your workout.

If you fancy just getting away from it all and escaping your thoughts, why not buy or make your own music compilation to keep you motivated and energised during your walking sessions (see page 51)?

Make sure you've an eye to safety at all times, especially if walking on your own. Go out in daylight or if you are out in the evening keep to busy, well-lit areas.

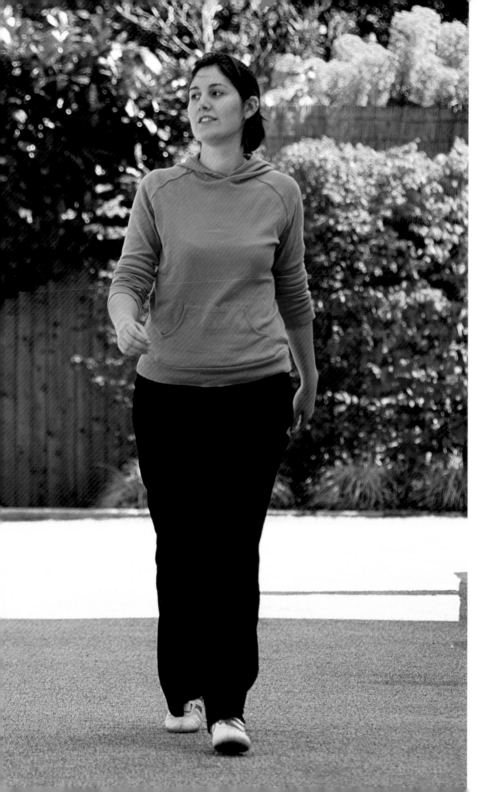

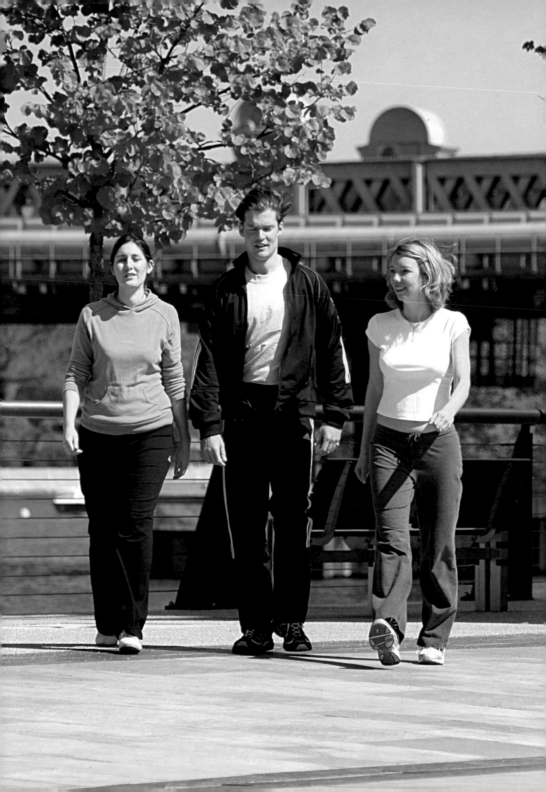

Walking with others

Walking is the perfect social activity, allowing people to improve their health and fitness while being able to chat and laugh with each other at the same time. Unlike other sports and activities, almost anyone can take part in a walk, so no-one need feel left out.

Bear in mind when walking in a group that the pace will be dictated by the least able member of the group. If you are going out for a social amble, then this might not matter. If you are walking for fitness, however, it's best if everyone in the group is of a similar fitness level so that you can all benefit from a proper workout.

There are plenty of ways in which to enjoy walking with a group:

► Get a group of friends together and go on a mystery tour! Meet at a train station and travel to a destination you are unfamiliar with to explore a new area.
► Incorporate a walk into the schedule of an event such as a conference or village fête.
► Or how about starting up a walking club ...

CASE STUDY **Amy (45)**

I feel much lighter and happier now. The WOW! Plan is great and I couldn't have done this on my own. I have met lots of new friends and now eat more healthily. I also choose to exercise now, going for walks at least twice a week.

Starting your own walking club

It can be fun to make your walking a social, team-building activity. Walking clubs have been around for many years all over the world. Why not start one yourself? You will be surprised at the level of interest you'll get – people are always looking for opportunities to meet and spend time with positive and like-minded individuals.

Why not ask around, put posters up or send emails to gauge interest. You could start one:

▶ Among your friends – ask each person to bring someone outside your circle along so you can all meet both old faces and new.
▶ At your workplace – colleagues may well be looking to do something healthy in their lunch break. Alternatively, you could set up a walk-to-work group, a great way to save money on transport while kick-starting your energy levels for a more productive and enjoyable day at the office.
▶ In your local neighbourhood – this is a great way to build community spirit and get to know the neighbours.
▶ To train for an event – maybe you could encourage a group to train for and take part in one of the many walking and running events around the world, from the local charity 5-mile walk/jog to the New York marathon. It will give you real purpose, an immense sense of achievement when you complete the course and, above all, you will reap enormous health and well-being benefits from becoming so fit.

Training for an event

There are thousands of events every year around the world that are based on either running or walking a certain distance. Often people take part for charity, raising sponsorship from friends, family and colleagues, while others participate for the sheer pleasure and satisfaction of pushing themselves to complete a set goal.

Whether you have entered a 5-km (3-mile) race or a marathon, you will need to prepare your body by following a suitable training programme. Below are some general tips to help you on your way:

NB The event organisers can often help you with your training programme so do ask for their advice and any information they can provide.

- ▶ Practise the WOW! walking techniques on a regular basis. This will aid your training programme and make you stronger and fitter than if you were to rely on normal walking alone.
- ▶ Depending on the distance of the event you have entered, you will need to increase your endurance, strength and speed. Be sure to include walks of varying distances and speed throughout the week (4 or 5 days), and factor in 2 or 3 recovery days to allow your body to repair itself.
- ▶ Include hills and stairs in your training to build up your strength. This will help you become resistant to injury and soreness, especially when walking on hard surfaces such as roads.
- ▶ When training seriously for an event, it is important to eat the right food and at the right time. Aim to keep your blood sugar levels as even as possible to prevent peaks and troughs in your energy levels and subsequent cravings for quick fixes (see page 59).
- ▶ Enjoy building your fitness and working towards your goals!

Motivation

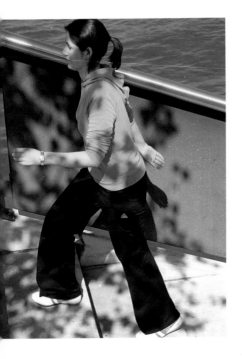

You know what you want to achieve, you've written down your goals and you're already seeing positive changes in your life. But we all experience a bit of a wobble from time to time. Perhaps things aren't going too well at work or there are problems at home and you have allowed these things to distract you.

The message is ... KEEP GOING

By sticking with The WOW! Plan and your new healthy habits, you will be far better able to cope with any problems that may arise in your life as a whole. If you persist and let nothing get in the way of your new healthy and positive attitude, you will succeed in this and in other areas of your life.

If you're having trouble sticking to your plan, here are some ideas to help you get back on track:

► Imagine yourself completing a good workout and focus on how great you'll feel at the end of it.
► Make regular exercise times and keep to them. Ensure that exercise is one of your top priorities every day.
► Give yourself a change. If you get tired of doing the same walk every day, choose a different route. Variety is the key to keeping you motivated – you'll find you look forward to different scenery.
► Take time out in the morning to exercise. Not only will you feel

energised for the rest of the day, but all day long you'll be burning more calories!

▶ Focus on how well you're doing an exercise rather than on just doing it. In this way you'll have greater success in sticking with it.

▶ Find walking buddies. Having people to work out with is a great motivation. You'll keep each other going and will be less likely to quit early.

▶ Take every opportunity to walk. Being active still counts, even if it's not a dedicated workout. Walk to the shop, take the stairs instead of the lift, walk during your lunch hour, etc.

▶ Log your walking with the Health Bank (see page 56). It helps you see how well you're doing and can encourage you to set new goals.

▶ Take the kids or the dog with you. If they rely on you for their daily dose of fresh air, you'll have an added reason to go out.

▶ Give yourself a reward for getting through it.

▶ Set-backs will happen... so just accept it. Don't let them get you down. Be determined and get right back to your routine.

▶ Focus on your progress. Remind yourself how much you have achieved since you started your new healthy lifestyle and remember the things that got you motivated in the first place.

▶ Smiling is proven to release 'the happy hormone', which should encourage you from within to do something positive. There are endless things in the world that can make you smile.

▶ Keep a favourite quote in your head. Look on the internet for one that works for you or use one of these:

'If you knew you could not fail, what would you do?'

'Everything is possible. You can achieve anything you set your mind to.'

'When the going gets tough, the tough get going – and that's me!'

Index